FOOD MATTERS

FOOD MATTERS

THE ROLE YOUR DIET PLAYS IN THE FIGHT AGAINST CANCER

DR SHUBHAM PANT

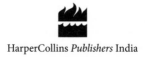

HarperCollins *Publishers* India

First published by HarperCollins *Publishers* in 2020
A-75, Sector 57, Noida, Uttar Pradesh 201301, India
www.harpercollins.co.in

2 4 6 8 10 9 7 5 3 1

P-ISBN: 978-93-9035-146-6
E-ISBN: 978-93-9035-143-5

Typeset in 11/14.8 Arno Pro at
Manipal Technologies Limited, Manipal

Printed and bound at
Replika Press Pvt. Ltd.

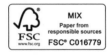

To my rays of sunshine, Anya and Shreya

And to patients and their caregivers

Contents

SECTION III
Surviving Cancer

Author's Note

I learned that every mortal will taste death. But only some will taste life.

—RUMI

'What do you mean you don't know which muscles attach to the knee joint?'

My father was trying hard to control the look of exasperation on his face. He was speaking calmly, but it was clear to an independent observer that he was in shock, disbelief, or both, at the same time. Emotions were running high in our house. It was a week before the 'Pre-Profs' or the preparatory examinations that are held in medical schools all around India before the dreaded 'Professionals' (end of semester exams). Some people want to get a 'D' (Distinction) whereas for the mere mortals it was about scraping through with a 'd' (dhakka; just above passing grade).

A little family background to explain this reaction. My father (Col. C.S. Pant, VSM) is a self-made man (the youngest of seven brothers) who in his twenties, as a young doctor in the Army, was posted with the Gurkha Rifles battalion on the frontlines of the 1971 war. Staffed only with two nursing assistants, he evacuated at least 50 wounded soldiers, hence playing a crucial role in lives saved. A radiologist by profession, he has co-authored several books and served as the president of the Indian Radiological Imaging Association. My mother was a physician in the Central Government Health Services who initially was accepted to a coveted residency in PGIMER Chandigarh but could not pursue it on account of family reasons. My sister… Where do I begin? First in class in her school since kindergarten and managed to clear both medical entrance exams and secure an admission to Economics Honours in St. Stephen's College, Delhi, which is no mean achievement.

Me … I was on a different trajectory. I still remember, in class 12, my mother had to come to pick me up from an inter-high school competition. Instead of going to my biology tuition, I had snuck away to help backstage at my school play.

However, by some strange twist of fate, I cleared the DPMT (or the Delhi University Pre-Medical Test) and gained admission to Maulana Azad Medical College (MAMC) in New Delhi. The first few years in medical school were a blur. No better way to excite an 18-year-old about the human anatomy than by exposing them to a corpse preserved in formalin that 30 eager students are crowding around, scalpels at the ready. Scaphoid, lunate, triquetral, pisiform, trapezium, trapezoid, capitate and hamate—who thought that one could have so many bones in one's wrist. And then to remember the entire sequence!

After the first few years that are non-clinical, you move into the clinical rotations where you see patients for the first time. That is when one steps out of a protective bubble into the harsh reality of life in India. Patients and families from all over flock to tertiary-care hospitals like the ones affiliated with MAMC, desperately hoping to save their loved ones. The overall experience was truly overwhelming and is akin to riding a roller-coaster with no breaks.

The OPD (outpatient department) consisted of a small windowless room with two desks where the interns (bottom feeders of the medical food chain) and residents (senior to the interns, but pretty much the lowest people on the totem pole) used to sit with a crush of patients coming in from all directions. Outside the room we had our friendly guard desperately trying (with very little success) to corral the crush of humanity in a line. One sees life, death, despair and hope within the span of an hour.

The inpatient wards were large halls with beds lined up, the lingering smell of phenyl in the air. But it was the pediatric wards that had the most profound effect on me. Family members bring their children from interior villages once they have exhausted all options. They worked their way through the village doctor, local 'specialist', district hospital and then to the place of last resort—the tertiary care center, many at death's doors. I can never forget the 'diarrhoea' ward where malnourished children with sunken sockets and protruding ribs struggled to stay alive even as their distraught parents watched over them. Along with the despair there was always the glimmer of hope. Children who looked like they had hours to live, started to run and talk after they were hydrated, and their dysentery subsided. The sparkle came back in the eyes of parents who had all but given up.

The experience of being in medical school is one of being a soldier in the battlefield: you try to dodge all the minefields, duck when bombs are tossed mercilessly at you (the endless examinations) and try to make it on the other side with life and limb intact. And finally … at the end, you are reminded of one the famous Murphy's laws: The light at the end of the tunnel … is the headlight of an oncoming train … The Intern Year (Remember: BOTTOM FEEDERS)!!!

Berthold Auerbach, the German poet, once said, 'Music washes away from the soul the dust of everyday life.' This was true for me as music was my escape from my Zombie-like sleep-deprived intern years. From concerts, festivals to listening to classic rock at a Delhi hang-out in New Friends Colony called the Mezz (people coming of age in Delhi in the 1990s might recognize this place), there was seldom a day without music. To pursue my interest, I auditioned for and was selected as a radio jockey by All India Radio to host the 'Western Music section' (this predates the FM stations of today). Along with my hospital duties, I was soon playing classic rock in shows like the Wicked Hour (from 1 a.m to 2 a.m which worked perfectly with my work schedule). It was an amazing time; for a couple of hours in the studio, I could kick back, relax, forget the day's grind and hang out with my friends The Doors, Deep Purple, Queen, The Eagles, Led Zeppelin, to name a few. Music was truly healing for my soul. But as they say, all good things must come to an end and I left to pursue my first love: of being a physician.

From my early days in medical school, I was fascinated by the field of cancer. My father's radiology clinic in Delhi was and is still dedicated to the early detection of breast cancer. I remember him patiently, and with great empathy, discussing with distraught patients and their families the diagnosis of cancer and guiding them through the next steps in dealing with a cancer diagnosis. I was always amazed at the fortitude of the patients, many of whom took the diagnosis in their stride and focused on the path ahead. I remember the case of a young lady, in her early thirties with two young children, who was diagnosed with breast cancer. She dealt with adversity like a champ, took matters in her own hands, shaved off her head and was a radiantly positive person, even through tough times. When I asked her if the loss of hair had been hard, she mentioned that it gave her a new look like Sinead O'Connor! (Again, for my '90s gang.) At that point in time, being a typical college kid, I was fretting over something unimportant, when her attitude towards her challenging situation completely blew my mind. I realized that my so-called 'struggles' were inconsequential; it gave me a different outlook, to not sweat the little things in life. To achieve my goal of specializing in oncology, I left for the US where I pursued a residency in Internal Medicine followed by a fellowship in my chosen specialty of Hematology-Oncology.

Cancer is a truly life-changing diagnosis which can take a physical, mental and economical toll. We normally take the simple things in life, like the ability to relish and taste our food, for granted … until it gets taken away from us. Patients who could eat a 10-course meal struggle to get a small morsel of food down. Taste buds go for a toss and things that were appetizing become repulsive overnight. Many patients develop a metallic taste, losing the ability to distinguish salt, sugar or both. People who were the epitome of health wither on account of the cancer or side effects of therapy.

I always get asked: How do you do this job and keep smiling; is it not depressing? I remember an incident, early on in my professional life when, on a visit to Delhi, I had a chance meeting with one of my friend's mothers who—like all helpful, Indian aunties—asked me what I was doing in America. When I told her that I was pursuing a career in cancer care, she looked at me quizzically, sighed and said, 'Why are you doing something so depressing, could you not get a fellowship in cardiology?' (That was a nice way of saying

I wasn't smart enough to study cardiology and had to settle for second-third best!).

Oncology for me is a truly rewarding profession as you get to interact and learn from patients and their caregivers who are at a very challenging time in their lives. Personally, taking care of patients has been immensely rewarding and has afforded me a unique perspective on life. I am reminded every day of the true wealth in life which is one's health. However tough the day, I know there are patients in the hospital who have struggles that dwarf any of my concerns. I savour the little things, like sitting outside when it's cold with a blanket, sipping a cup of tea, singing loudly in the car when my favourite song comes on the radio, vegging on the couch with the family, reciting a prayer with my daughter at bedtime. I enjoy the mundane. I am often reminded of the lesson 'In Celebration of Being Alive' I read as part of my English course in school. This centered around the experience of Dr Christiaan Barnard, a South African cardiac surgeon, who performed the world's first human-to-human heart transplant in 1967. Per the story, Dr Barnard was rounding in the hospital one day when he saw two children suffering from terminal illnesses racing on an unattended breakfast trolley in the hospital. One was a 'driver' and the other a 'mechanic'. The 'mechanic' was blind on account of suffering third-degree burns on the upper side of his body and the 'driver' had undergone an amputation for a malignant tumour. Inspite of these overwhelming odds, the children were determined to have fun and make the most out of life.

The children taught him an important lesson: no matter how hard our struggles in life, no matter how desperate the situation, we should try to cherish and live each day ... in celebration of being alive.

Introduction

Out of clutter, find simplicity.

—ALBERT EINSTEIN

At 35 years of age, I realized that something was amiss. I was always a scrawny, underweight kid, but age was rapidly catching up and I was caught unawares. No longer could I gulp down sodas, gorge on sweets and ice-cream everyday and not see the 'side' effects. First, I was in denial. My waist size increased and so did the size of my trousers. I used to drive by gymnasiums, but never make it in. Tried to eat healthy but lasted only a few days (seemed like months!). I took to watching workout videos to motivate myself, but the only part of my body that exercised was my eyes. Sounds familiar?

The turning point came when I was months away from my 36th birthday and we were expecting our second daughter. It struck me that it was now or never. I walked into that gym and have never walked out. I always used to talk to my patients about a healthy diet, but now I began practicing what I preached and started my own journey with health and healing. I lost 20 kilos and about five inches from my waist. I started researching more about diet and its impact on the human body and the lesson I learnt is that when it comes to cancer, complexity is the norm, not the exception.

This helped me grow as a physician, because as an oncologist, I was often asked, 'Doctor, what can I do or eat to decrease my risk of cancer?' both in professional settings and at casual gatherings. Nutrition and diet become even more critical for patients diagnosed with cancer, but unfortunately, this aspect is put on the backburner and is seldom addressed during or after cancer therapy. The chasm is often filled by 'miracle cures' and 'food fads' that frequently hurt more than help. The more I discussed with patients and families, I realized that there existed a need to empower patients, caregivers and healthcare workers to incorporate nutrition to maintain health and well-being alongside their therapy.

To understand the complex interplay between diet and exercise, it is important to understand how cancer develops. Cancer is caused when regular cells go rogue. Think of the human body as a well-tuned assembly line where every cell is checked for deformities by the body's immune system. If a cell is not behaving itself, then it gets taken off the assembly line and it is discarded, a process called cell death or 'apoptosis'. Unfortunately, sometimes the cell undergoes a mutation and transforms, so the body's defense mechanisms fail to recognize it and the cell grows unchecked and eventually develops into cancer. Mutations can increase when there is chronic inflammation in the body.

While there are certain factors like genetics and, to an extent, environment that you cannot control, there are others like diet and lifestyle that are controllable factors. For example, placing tobacco between cheek and gum or teeth for long periods can lead to chronic inflammation in the oral mucosa and increase the risk of cancer of the mouth. Similarly, when one is obese, the body is in constant stress and that creates a low level of chronic inflammation that, in turn, can lead to adverse outcomes. Food through a healthy diet rich in vegetables, whole grains and whole fruits can help the body's repair mechanisms and fix some of the damage. On the other hand, increased consumption of an excess amount of red meat and processed meats has the potential to increase the cancer risk.

Bottom line is that what you eat can have a long-term impact on your health and well-being including chronic illnesses like heart disease and cancer.

Unfortunately, with the advent the 24/7 news cycle, 'click-bait' headlines are everywhere, but evidence which is dependable and science-based guidelines is hard to find. The best way to determine if an intervention is working is to conduct a randomized controlled trial in which participants are 'randomized' by chance to one intervention or another. One of the first randomized trials carried out was by James Lind who was a physician in the royal navy in the 1700s. At that time scurvy (due to a deficiency of vitamin C) was very common amongst sailors on ships who were at sea for months on end. Back then, the concept of vitamins was unknown, and Lind thought that scurvy was due to 'putrefaction' of the body and could be helped by acids. He thus chose to include a dietary supplement of an acidic quality in the experiment. He 'randomized' twelve sailors with scurvy in six groups of two each. All of them received the same diet, but in addition group one was given a quart of cider daily, group two 25 drops of elixir of vitriol (sulfuric acid), group three six spoonfuls of vinegar, group four half a pint of seawater, group five received two oranges and one lemon (my guess is the people he liked the most!), and the last group a spicy paste plus a drink of barley water (people he liked the least!). The treatment of group five stopped after six days when they ran out of fruit, but by that time one sailor was fit for duty while the other had almost recovered. Thus, it could be hypothesized that citrus fruits seemed to have an effect on scurvy.

More than two hundred years after the James Lind experiment, Jules Hirsch, a physician scientist at The Rockefeller University helped clarify some of the prevailing misconceptions about obesity with his research. In the 1980s, Hirsch and his colleagues studied 41 volunteers, 18 of whom were obese and 23 who had never been overweight. All participants were admitted to the hospital and fed a liquid diet, first up to 6,000 extra calories daily until they gained 10 per cent of their normal weight and then decreasing it down to 800 calories each day to lose weight. The researchers found that when the participants' weight increased so did the rate of metabolism; when they returned to their basal weights, their rates of metabolism also dropped to what they had been at the start. Interestingly, as the subjects dropped weight, their energy expenditure decreased to amounts greater than could be accounted for by the loss of body mass, i.e., their metabolism slowed down considerably. Hence this provided a biological explanation for what you may have experienced—it is hard to lose weight but it is even harder to keep it off!

As these controlled studies can be extremely challenging to conduct in the general population, many nutrition studies rely on food surveys, so called M-BM (memory-based dietary assessment methods). In this, the scientists ask a group of study participants, often referred to as a cohort, what they ate, their habits (smoking, alcohol use, etc.). The participants then are tracked over time to see if they developed any health conditions like cancer.

The problem is that in real life it is extremely challenging to accurately recount what we had for breakfast that day, leave alone a few days or a week back. Try this experiment: Close your eyes and try and remember what you had for lunch yesterday in granular detail. How much rice did you have: one cup or two cups, did you apply butter, what about vegetables and salad, what was the exact quantity? Kudos to you if you can accurately answer these questions. Now think about what you had a week back … any luck? Other than the gifted few, if you are like me, it is truly a herculean task to remember what EXACTLY you ate a few days ago in minute detail. Hence, it is challenging to accurately quantify the effect of specific foods based on these surveys.

However, it is possible for you to cut through the omnipresent background noise and make healthy diet and lifestyle decisions. When evaluating studies in humans, the focus should be on the cumulative research (clinical trials, cohort studies, systematic reviews, meta-analysis) instead of studies that cannot be replicated. Prospective cohort studies which follow participants from exposure (e.g., smoking) to the occurrence of the disease (e.g. lung cancer) require long-term follow-up and even with their shortcomings, can be useful. Multiple studies, with a majority pointing in the same direction, can give one reasonable confidence about the link between a diet and a disease like cancer. Exercise caution and be very careful before making drastic lifestyle decisions based on single studies, especially those that make tall unsubstantiated claims.

The link between diet and cancer is complicated and most of the research points to an association, but it cannot be said with certainty that one kind of food will help prevent cancer. But certain dietary choices and patterns can help in decreasing the risk. The science of nutrition is multifaceted and it is important to be a critical thinker and learn how to interpret results for yourself, to make appropriate dietary choices.

SECTION I

Diet and Cancer Prevention

An ounce of prevention is worth a pound of cure.

—BENJAMIN FRANKLIN

1

India: We Have a Problem

I was enjoying a peaceful dinner at a family friend's house when a well-meaning 'Scotched-up' uncle plonked down on the sofa next to me and began chatting: So, young man, what do you do? I went in to my usual 'Standard Operating Procedure' response about being a cancer doctor, etc. And then came the barrage of questions: Why did I think everyone in India was getting cancer? How does cancer really develop? What should be done to avoid it? Before I could say anything, he proclaimed he already knew the answers, as someone had recently shared some illuminating forwards on his WhatsApp group. The rest of what he said was a blur of generic statements, apparently validated by a very famous 'university' in the States. Before I could counter him, he left saying he wanted to head outside for a smoke. The irony was not lost on me.

Cancer: It's Everywhere!

So, what's really going on in India? Over 61 per cent of total deaths in India are attributed to lifestyle or non-communicable diseases. India has an estimated 22.2 million Chronic Obstructive Pulmonary Disease (COPD) patients and 35 million chronic asthma patients. Twenty-six per cent deaths in India occur due to cardiovascular diseases. Unfortunately, cancer is contributing to this trend with an estimated 6,00,000–7,00,000 cancer-related deaths in 2012.[1] From 1990 to 2016, cancer has jumped from seventh position to fourth position in causes of most number of deaths in the country, with an increase in the incidence in states all over India (**Figure 1**). This number is continuing to increase steeply and it is expected that 1.73 million new cancer cases will likely be recorded by 2020. The geography of cancer in India is varied, with more cases of gall bladder cancer in north India than stomach cancer in the south.

Nowadays, it is not uncommon to know someone who has received a diagnosis of cancer which was rare in the '80s and nineties, when I was growing up in Delhi. The cause for this increase is multifactorial and cannot be explained in a few 'clickbait' headlines. A major avoidable cause, however, is lack of knowledge. Cancer in India is increasingly associated with use of tobacco products; indoor and outdoor pollution; infections such as Human papillomavirus, Hepatitis B, and Helicobacter pylori; low screening; early detection; and possibly diet and sedentary lifestyles. As an example, in the year 2016–2017, 19 per cent of men, 2 per cent of women and 10 per cent (99.5 million) of all adults smoked tobacco; 29.6 per cent of men, 12.8 per cent of women and 21.4 per cent (199.4 million) adults used smokeless tobacco. A whopping 298.9 million of all adults used tobacco (smoked and/or smokeless tobacco)! When asked, 92.4 per cent of these adults believed that smoking did indeed cause serious illnesses and about 95.6 per cent believed that the use of smokeless tobacco causes serious illnesses—still, they continued to indulge in this dangerous habit. In 2020, air pollution, tobacco, alcohol and diet changes are the primary triggers of cancer.

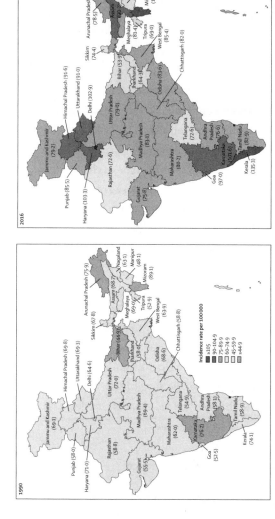

Figure 1: The burden of cancers and their variations across the states of India: the Global Burden of Disease Study 1990–2016.*

* 'The burden of cancers and their variations across the states of India: the Global Burden of Disease Study 1990–2016', *Lancet Oncol*, 2018; 19: 1289–306, https://creativecommons.org/licenses/by/4.0/.# The states of Chhattisgarh, Jharkhand, Telangana, and Uttarakhand did not exist in 1990, as they were created from existing larger states in 2000 or later. Data for these four new states were disaggregated from their parent states based on their current district composition. These states are shown in the 1990 map for comparison with 2016.

Ironically, one of the main reasons for the increase in incidence of cancer is the dark lining to the silver cloud of improved lifespan. Confused? Let me explain. While many understand the gravity of the disease, not many grasp the biological mechanism of the disease. Life expectancy in India has risen from 41 years in 1960 to 69 years in 2015, with it being as high as 75 years in states like Kerala. This has been possible on account of improvements in sanitation and a decrease in deaths due to infectious disease, as was common before. Though we hear about young people developing cancer, the vast majority of cancers are diagnosed after the age of 55, so the longer we live, the more our chances of developing cancer. Cancer starts at the microscopic level, when a cell undergoes a change or a mutation. The human body is unique and is composed of trillions of cells undergoing division at all time. Think of our body as a massive, but fine-tuned assembly line. Each time a part becomes defective, it is either fixed or removed. In a similar fashion, when a cell in our body starts misbehaving, the human body either corrects the defect or the cell dies, a process called apoptosis. However, as we age, this machinery becomes defective and the cells with the mutation go rogue and start dividing uncontrollably, leading to the development and spread of cancer. In short: cancer is complicated and is not one disease, it is a conglomeration of more than a hundred different diseases that cannot be targeted by a single 'magic bullet'. However, there are avoidable lifestyle changes that we can make to decrease the risks of contracting this dreaded disease.

The Rise of Social Media: The Death of Science

So, how was the uncle at the dinner so confident of himself? Two words: social media. I would be lying if I told you I am not guilty of spending more time on social media than any reasonable person should. How could taking out a few minutes (or hours) out of our productive time to catch up on cat videos, good morning messages or what latest party we were not invited to be a negative influence on us? Though social media may serve as a place where one keeps in touch with friends and family, these platforms are a cesspool of disinformation, especially when it comes to complicated diseases like cancer. It is not uncommon to get forwards, especially in family groups, that 'inform' people about the latest health trend, or new medical research or home remedies that will cure cancer, diabetes, and many other ailments. These social media forwards became so prevalent and gathered such a following that it became imperative to inform people to not trust everything they read on their phone screens. For example, in 2018, no sooner had a well-known Bollywood actress come out with her cancer diagnosis than the following message started making rounds on chat groups:

Kick off 'Breast Cancer'... Avoid black bra in summer, always cover your chest completely with your dupatta or scarf when you are under the sun...Pass it to All the Ladies you Care for without hesitation.

The forward was soon, thankfully, marked as 'fake'.

Such false information can be easily disseminated in India, where there are reported to be more than 500 million (50 crore) smartphone users in 2019, according to a market research firm techARC report. A massive section of society now relies on consuming news and entertainment through a mobile device and is bombarded by news which is hard to verify as real or fake. As per the website, Check4Spam.com, 25 per cent of fake messages can relate to 'medical advice', where 'medical cures' are sold to patients with cancer who are most vulnerable. The post below (**Figure 2**) is an example of the misinformation spread on social media:

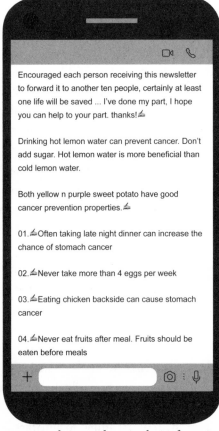

Figure 2: Chat groups are being used to spread misinformation about cancer.

Take a minute to read through these messages, and deconstruct the advice given here. It is clear that these are just random statements without any proof or data backing them up. Some posts even say 'as recommended by (some famous institute)' without a link to the data or the research behind it. There are also self-styled 'health gurus' who readily give advice on everything from how to keep your hair healthy to more dangerous and potentially harmful advice on how to cure cancer. When it comes to your health, be a champion for yourself and be careful where you get your advice from, as an innocuous statement can lead to long-term and permanent harm for your body.

Social media can serve as an echo chamber where one goes to affirm one's already held views. Internet activist Eli Pariser coined a phrase to denote the practice of algorithmic editing by companies to show individuals the information they agree with, while filtering out opposing views: the filter bubble. This can increase the possibility of interpreting facts to confirm our beliefs, a phenomenon called confirmation bias, and it is getting more commonplace. For example, in his book *Research in Psychology: Methods and Design*, C. James Goodwin gives an example of confirmation bias as it applies to extrasensory perception:

> Persons believing in extrasensory perception (ESP) will keep close track of instances when they were 'thinking about Mom, and then the phone rang and it was her!' Yet they ignore the far more numerous times when (a) they were thinking about Mom and she didn't call and (b) they weren't thinking about Mom and she did call. They also fail to recognize that if they talk to Mom about every two weeks, their frequency of 'thinking about Mom' will increase near the end of the two-week-interval, thereby increasing the frequency of a 'hit'.[2]

I want you to think about the last time you were on a search engine trying to confirm news that deep down you already agree with. Chances are, you kept scrolling till you found a story which affirms your already held belief: sounds familiar? It is a telling sign of the times when both the American Dialect Society and Collins English Dictionary named 'fake news' as its word of the year for 2017.

This can, however, easily snowball into real world medical consequences. It is commonplace for headings like 'Ten Cancer-Causing Foods You Should Stop Eating Today' followed by one-liners which link the food to a chemical (which may be present in minute quantities) and declare it to be a 'cancer causing food'. It is also commonplace to get emails and forwards which proclaim: 'Eat This Superfood to Prevent Cancer' with a 'helpful' link to where you can procure this food. Without confirmation, individuals end up sharing it, leading to a cascade effect where no one bothers to check the source. A commentary in 2013 by Maki Inoue-Choi, an epidemiologist at the National Cancer Institute, described an example of an episode on the *Dr Oz Show* that suggested an endive (a leaf vegetable similar to lettuce) was an 'anti-cancer' food that can decrease the risk of ovarian cancer by 75 per cent. The miraculous agent in endive–kaempferol– had demonstrated in laboratory experiments that it might have some properties curbing unchecked growth of cells; however, it was unclear if this would help with regular dietary intake. This apparent 'association' was in only one study and the authors found no link with ovarian cancer risk when they evaluated other foods that provided more kaempferol per serving than endive[3]. Per the authors, 'Media coverage of these so-called "miracle foods" is often just a marketing tool. Stories of "miracle foods" sell magazines and advertising space; food industries often sponsor research to show that their foods or products are superior, and supplement industries look to boost sales. In real life, however, we do not live on one single food item. We eat meals that consist of a considerable variety of foods, several times each day.'

We all need to be better watchdogs and always check the source of dietary advice floating about and share information only if we know it is from a reputable source. Beware of headlines which scream 'breakthrough', 'miracle' or 'cure' and make sure you don't just click the 'Like' or 'Share' button before you read the entire article and, if possible, go to the source of the article. A number of these studies are done using mice, but are projected as the next big thing and I think all of us can agree to the fact that mice are NOT men!!! Be aware of any attempt to distill the interplay of food and cancer in 280 characters, as when evaluating diet and cancer in the context of the human body, complexity is definitely the norm, not the exception.

What's (Indian) Food Got to Do with It?

India is the epitome of diversity, with distinct cultures and dietary preferences in each region. From the rotis in the north to fish in the east to sambhar, rasam, tamarind and curd of the south: there is truly unity in 'foodie' diversity. The traditional Indian diet already did incorporate the elements recommended by the American Cancer Society (ACS), which endorses a plant-based diet rich in fibre with at least 2.5 cups of vegetable or fruit a day and limits on the intake of red meat. However, an economic boom in the last two decades has resulted in rapid urbanization and an increase in disposable income, heralding a sea change in dietary and lifestyle habits. Processed eatables, including so-called 'junk foods', are making inroads into people's houses and appetites, along with an increase in tobacco (both smoking and smokeless) and alcohol consumption. This, coupled with increasingly sedentary lifestyles and a rise in obesity, has resulted in an explosion of various non-communicable diseases like cancer. Though there are a number of theories on why exactly a person develops cancer, there are lifestyle and diet modifications that can decrease one's risk of contracting the disease. Here's some food for thought: A staggering 30–40 per cent of cancers are preventable by healthy lifestyle choices such as avoidance of tobacco and public health measures like immunization against cancer causing infections.

The New 'Fast Food Nation'

I remember my idyllic upbringing in Delhi. My father was in the Armed Forces Medical Corps and I grew up as an Army brat living it up in the Delhi cantonment. It was an amazing childhood, we biked everywhere, in the club we swam (only on 'even' days—this was peculiar to the Dhaula Kuan club to decrease overcrowding in the pool. The ones whose membership number ended with an even number would get to swim on the even days in the month) and played tennis, spending most of our free time outdoors. Once in a blue moon, for a treat we would be taken out to Nirula's in Chanakyapuri, where we would gorge on the cheese sausage pizza and finish it off with a family-sized hot chocolate fudge. This was a treat that we looked forward to for months on end—this was an indulgence and not a daily routine. In college in the 1990s we first heard about a pizza chain coming to town and excitedly looked forward to the same. From 1995, when I entered college, to 2000, when I graduated, the whole food scene had been turned on its head. As the Western lifestyle paved its way into India along with rapid urbanization and higher disposable incomes, the Indian middle class experimented with this new trend, which is now a part of their lifestyle. With the introduction of mall culture and food courts, and their value-for-money pricing, hassle-free ways, and casual atmosphere, Indians started enjoying the idea of eating out. Gone were the mom and pop shops, replaced by glitzy, shiny uber-convenient fast food joints that drew in crowds by the hundreds. I still remember when McDonald's opened its first store in Vasant Vihar in Delhi: the line stretched on for blocks! Since then the fast food trend has been growing at breakneck speed: Taco Bell, Krispy Kreme, Burger King, Pizza Hut, Dunkin' Donuts, Domino's: you name it, we have it! As per a study done by analysts at Technopak, a management consulting firm in Gurgaon, the Indian market for chain restaurants was an estimated $2.5 billion in 2013 and is expected to grow to $8 billion in 2020, driven by the growth of what is known as quick-service, or fast food, restaurants.[4]

There is no doubt that India is in the midst of a rapid lifestyle transition with an exponential increase in poor dietary habits, obesity and inactive lifestyles. There is an 'obesity epidemic' and a 'nutrition transition', with the whole plant content of diets being replaced by processed foods, fried foods and refined carbohydrates.[5] This is particularly concerning for the next generation as the intake of processed foods is increasing among children. The Centre for Science and Environment, a Delhi-based research and advocacy organization, conducted a survey of over 13,000 children in the age group of 9–17 from 300 schools, a majority of them from urban areas. The results were startling as they showed that that 93 per cent of the children ate packaged foods, 68 per cent consumed sugar-sweetened beverages more than once a week, and 27 per cent ate at fast food outlets more than once a week.[6] This was at the cost of healthy foods like millets, fruits and vegetables which were consumed more sparingly than recommended for a healthy balanced diet.

In addition to the inroads made by fast food, features of the nutrition transition have included the use of white rice (dehusked and highly polished) instead of brown rice (unmilled, hand-pounded, parboiled rice which retains bran and germ components), substitution of lentils, fruits, vegetables, unrefined whole grains, nuts and seeds with refined carbohydrates and potatoes, hydrogenated oils (such as Vanaspati) and the increased intake of fast food. At the same time, unfortunately, the variety of grains in contemporary Indian diets has decreased, with whole grains such as barley, amaranth, and millet being sidelined for processed foods.[7] Recent research revealed that 50–60 per cent of total salt, sugar, and fat in Indian markets is procured by bulk purchasers to manufacture processed food items.[8] India is truly at the precipice of a lifestyle catastrophe with an increase in sedentary lifestyles and a rise in obesity, which is a risk factor for cancer. Fat density and total energy intake were associated with an increased risk of postmenopausal breast cancer, randomized tests by the Women's Health Initiative found, which was thought to be mediated by body fat deposition over time.[9] In contrast, traditional diets, which have high amounts of fruits and vegetables and are low in fat, have been associated with lower risk of breast cancer.[10] One of the major causes of concern is that not only is the obesity epidemic ravaging urban India, but is also emerging in rural India.[11]

The Real Secret to Decreasing Your Risk of Cancer

Picture this: a young attractive couple getting cosy on a bike, a polo player, numerous Bollywood actors looking cool; some ads telling us to 'Live Life Kingsize', or if you smoked a certain brand of cigarettes you were 'one of a kind'. And who can forget the ever-playing ad when the groom's parents pose a suggestion to the jittery prospective in-laws: 'Just greet us with paan masala.' The bride's father quickly brings out a can of paan masala—smiles all around! Heck, even the suave, bearded James Bond (aka Pierce Brosnan) was spotted with a box of paan masala and an advert touting 'Class never goes out of style' till he accused the company of 'unauthorized and deceptive use' of his image to endorse paan masala. He claimed that the contract said he was to advertise a 'breath freshener/tooth whitener'.

The campaign has been relentless and omnipresent and, unfortunately, it has worked. Though smoking is down in the West, countries in Asia have taken over the mantle, with China and India with the highest numbers of smokers worldwide, accounting for 307 million and 106 million respectively of the world's 1.1 billion adult smokers. In addition, India also has 200 million of the world's 367 million smokeless tobacco users.[12]

Per the WHO Global Adult Tobacco Survey 2016-2017[13], in India 19 per cent of men, 2 per cent of women and 10 per cent (99.5 million) of all adults smoked tobacco; 29.6 per cent of men, 12.8 per cent of women and 21.4 per cent (199.4 million) adults use smokeless tobacco. A whopping 266.8 million of all adults use tobacco (smoked and/or smokeless tobacco)! When asked, 92.4 per cent of these adults believed that smoking did indeed cause serious illnesses and about 95.6 per cent believed that the use of smokeless tobacco causes serious illnesses—still, they continued to indulge in this dangerous habit. Unfortunately, the risk was not only restricted to smokers. Thirty eight percent of adults were exposed to second hand smoke at home and 30.2 per cent adults who work indoors are exposed to second-hand smoke in the workplace.[14]

In addition to cigarettes and beedis, there are also major problems with smokeless tobacco, like betel quid and khaini, which is widely prevalent both in the urban and rural areas and is shockingly being used by children as young as fourteen years of age[15] (**Figure 3**). The National Family Health Survey showed that 21 per cent of people over 15 years of age consumed paan masala or tobacco. There are strict laws against tobacco in India, such as the Cigarettes and Other Tobacco Products Act 2003, but enforcement is remiss. In Mumbai, after the ban on paan masala and gutka, sales came down and the percentage of users quitting and reducing the habit was 23.53 per cent and 55.88 per cent respectively. The main reason of quitting and reduction in consumption was

Figure 3: Tobacco Products Commonly Used in India*

		ITEM	DESCRIPTION
• Smoked tobacco		Beedis	Sun dried and flaked tobacco wrapped in dried tendu leaves
		Chillum	A clay pipe used for smoking tobacco
		Hookah	Device used for vaporising and smoking flavoured tobacco. The vapour or smoke is passed through water before inhalation
		Cigarettes	A roll of cured and finely cut tobacco leaves and reconstituted tobacco rolled into a paper cylinder
		Cigars	Tightly rolled bundles of dried and fermented tobacco
		Chutta	Rolled tobacco leaves used like cigars
		Reverse chutta smoking or 'addapoga'	Smoking practice keeping the lighted end of the chutta in the mouth and inhaling it

		ITEM	DESCRIPTION
• Smoke-less tobacco	Oral form	Paan with tobacco	Paan consists of four main ingredients: betel leaf, areca nut (supari), slaked lime (chuna) and catechu, often consumed with tobacco
		Khaini	Crushed dried tobacco leaves mixed with slaked lime and chewed as a quid
		Gutkha	Preparation of crushed betel nut, tobacco, and sweet or savory flavorings, sold in small packets
		Paan masala	A commercial preparation of areca nut, slaked lime, catechu and condiments with or without powdered tobacco
		Gudaku, Mishri	Paste of tobacco and sugar molasses applied on gums Mishri — roasted tobacco powder applied as tooth powder
		Mawa	Combination of areca nut pieces, scented tobacco and slaked lime mixed on the spot and chewed
	Nasal form	Dry snuff	A small quantity of very fine tobacco powder mixed with aromatic substances inhaled through nose

*'Recognize Tobacco in its Many Forms', US Food and Drug Administration, 5 May 2016, https://www.fda.gov/consumers/consumer-updates/recognize-tobacco-its-many-forms

Chadda R., Sengupta S., 'Tobacco use by Indian adolescents', Tobacco Induced Diseases, 15 Jun 2002, 1(1):8-8, https://europepmc.org/article/pmc/2669568

'Commonly used smokeless tobacco products around the globe', WHO Framework Convention on Tobacco Control, https://untobaccocontrol.org/kh/smokeless-tobacco/paan-betel-quid-tobacco/

non-availability of these products. In spite of the ban, gutka was still available but in different forms or at an increased cost.

Amongst all that we have discussed, the most important intervention you can do to decrease your risk of developing cancer is to STOP using tobacco products. Tobacco contains at least 69 cancer causing chemicals in tobacco smoke and its use is the single largest preventable cause of cancer and is responsible for approximately 22 per cent of deaths from cancer worldwide.

Here's a common question that is often asked of me: My friend/neighbour used tobacco all their lives, but did not develop cancer and another person who never smoked was diagnosed with lung cancer. So why quit? Here's why: Though it is true that all tobacco users do not get cancer, the Centers for Disease Control and Prevention (CDC) notes that an active smoker's risk climbs with each year and with each cigarette smoked. For instance, if you smoke, you are 15 to 30 times likelier to develop lung cancer than if you don't. To make things worse, lung cancer is not the only thing you have to worry about—smoking can also cause cancers of the oesophagus, throat, mouth, kidney, bladder, liver, pancreas, stomach, cervix, colon, and rectum, as well as a blood cancer called Acute Myeloid leukemia. (**Figure 4**) Smoking not only harms you, it can harm people around you: it is estimated that living with a smoker increases a non-smoker's chances of developing lung cancer by 20 to 30 per cent.[16] There is no 'smoking occasionally'; no amount of smoking is safe. It includes all forms—cigars, hookahs, pipes—all of it. And remember: just because some marketing genius put 'light' or 'ultra light' in front of a product's name does not mean they are any safer for you; all cause harm.

Here is the good news: it is never too late to quit. Within five years of quitting smoking, the risk of cancers of the mouth, throat,

Figure 4: Tobacco use* causes cancer throughout the body

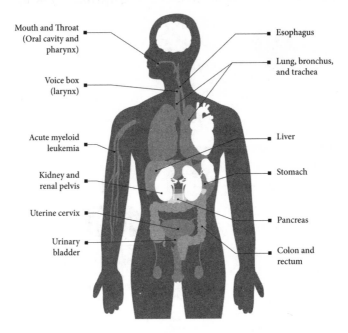

Mouth and Throat (Oral cavity and pharynx)

Esophagus

Lung, bronchus, and trachea

Voice box (larynx)

Acute myeloid leukemia

Liver

Kidney and renal pelvis

Stomach

Uterine cervix

Pancreas

Urinary bladder

Colon and rectum

* Includes both smoked (cigarettes, cigars) and smokeless (chewing tobacco, snuff) tobacco products that have been shown to cause cancer till date.

oesophagus, and bladder are cut in half and the cervical cancer risk falls to that of a non-smoker. The cherry on top is that your body begins to heal in a matter of a few minutes after quitting, and the benefits are life-long, as is evidenced in Figure 5. To my hipster friends: You can do all the yoga you want and eat organic, consume all the acai berries, and drink all the pomegranate juice you can lay your hands on. But if you smoke or chew tobacco, you are exponentially increasing your risk of cancer and have embarked on a dangerous journey that can result in catastrophic consequences.[17]

Figure 5: The Health Benefits of Quitting Smoking

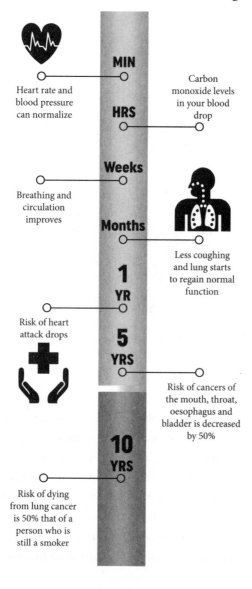

2

Food: It's Complicated

The Etymology of the word 'food' is thought to be from an old Germanic verb *fodjan*, which means 'to feed.' Food is called by a number of names depending on geography, including 'khana' in Hindi, 'Comida' in Spanish and 'Aliments' in French. Recently, though a number of pre-fixes have been added to the 'humble' food in an effort to make it more 'sexier' and palatable (pun intended!).

Case in point is a food fad that has emerged in the past decade: the so-called 'superfoods'. From the terminology, it seems like these are better and have special powers (like superman/woman) than the usual, run-of-the-mill 'non-superfoods'. They are supposed to be the magic elixir to combat all diseases: cardiac, cancer, even stress! The focus is on single nutrients or 'superfoods' to fight cancer. There are ads all over television and on the web promoting the 'health and cancer-fighting' benefits of a juice, shake or some obscure fruit from the Amazon jungle. I Googled the term 'superfoods and cancer' and got 11,700,000 results and everything—from tomatoes and broccoli to apricot beans and sprouted moong beans to the more exotic camu camu—all make the list in various online forums. The issue is, there is really no standard nutrition definition of what qualifies as a 'superfood', so the definition is open to interpretation. In fact, the very concept is thought by many to be a marketing tool. In 2007, EU legislation banned the use of the term superfood unless it was accompanied by a specific authorized health claim that explained to consumers why the product is good for their health. Now, don't get me wrong: I love blueberries as much as the next person and some foods do possess certain characteristics that would make them a healthier alternative. However, one should look at food in its entirety, and not rely on a few stand-alone sexy, in-style vegetables or fruits. (**Figure 6**)

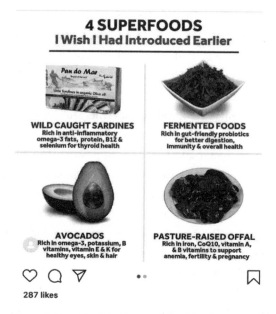

Figure 6: Superfoods is a buzzword and is often touted as miracle food.

In this world of constantly changing food trends and background noise, it is important to remember that diet and exercise, partly through their ability to influence body weight and prevent obesity, are increasingly recognized as important determinants of human cancer risk.[18] Nutrition plays an important role in cancer prevention[19]. The components of our daily diet have the ability to influence several processes that are important in the formation of cancer cells.[20] They can impact processes of inflammation, the immune system, regulation of hormones in the body, repair of DNA—all which can influence the development of cancer.[21]

To reiterate: no single food can help prevent chronic diseases. Rather, we have to be holistic in our approach and look at the overall diet rather than any single nutrient. To put it simply, look at your nutrition journey as a movie and DO NOT be fooled by the trailer! Be consistent and make incorporating healthy foods into your meals a habit, as your grandmother probably told you. So the next time you shop for 'superfoods' in the grocery store, give some love to 'non-superfoods', like the apple. Don't you think it deserves as much attention as the 'cool' blueberries?

Eat This...

Superfoods aside, the ACS guidelines for a healthy diet advocate what is easily achievable through an Indian diet. The recommendations emphasize plant-based foods with at least 2.5 cups of vegetable and fruits daily while limiting the intake of red meat (such as pork, lamb) and processed meats (hot dogs, sausages). Here's the good news: traditional Indian diets already incorporate the elements that the ACS recommends, a plant-based diet that is fibre rich. Dietary fibre has been linked to a lower risk of some types of cancer, especially colorectal cancer. The 'bad' and the 'ugly' of it is, over the past decades, we have moved away from traditional foodgrains, that actually were healthy, to eating polished, less nutritious alternatives.

Make Whole Grains Sexy Again: Time to Head Back to Our Roots

The Green Revolution in India was adopted by the Indian government in the 1960s to decrease the dependence on foreign foodgrains and increase the production of high-yield crops. Before the change in farming practices, traditional meals were derived from wholegrain carbohydrates including amaranth, barley, millet, and other ancient grains that have been grown on the Indian subcontinent for hundreds of years.[22] Though it did lead to food security and prosperity at first, there were some unintended consequences. The overwhelming increase in farming over the years, combined with increasing reliance on pesticides and fertilizers and an ever-shrinking water table, led to degradation of the fragile ecosystem. This also led to the shift from traditional foodgrains to refined grains. Refined grains such as white rice and refined wheat flour becoming staples in the Indian diet is a relatively recent change if you take into account hundreds of years of traditional practice. Early diets emphasized cereals, brown rice, pulses, roots, and tubers, and curd as a protein source.[23] The Indian diet is high in carbohydrates (70–80 per cent of total daily caloric intake) and low in protein (9–10 per cent of total daily caloric intake) which is lower than the recommendations by the Indian Council of Medical Research (60 per cent carbohydrate, 10–12 per cent protein).[24] Unfortunately, unlike ancient India, the overall variety of grains used in modern Indian diets is greatly reduced, with whole grains high in protein and fibre no longer contributing to the diet.[25] For example, a study conducted in Chennai found that nearly half of daily energy intake came from refined grains, and that white polished rice constituted 75 per cent of refined grain intake.[26] This is concerning as data from the Nurse's Health Study and the Health Professional's Follow-Up Study suggests that substitution of brown rice for white rice was associated with a lower risk of type 2 diabetes.[27]

The ancient grains also have traditionally a low glycaemic index, which is associated with numerous health benefits. The glycaemic index is a relative ranking of carbohydrate in foods according to how they affect blood glucose levels. Carbohydrates with a low glycaemic index are more slowly digested, absorbed, and metabolized and cause a lower and slower rise in blood glucose and, therefore, insulin levels. In contrast, foods like white bread and polished white rice are absorbed and converted into sugar rapidly in the blood, spiking insulin.

A great example is finger millet, also known as red millet, caracan millet, koracan, or ragi.[28] It has been an important staple food in India for generations.[29] It is grown and consumed throughout the country, from Uttarakhand in the north to Tamil Naidu in the south. Finger millet has a number of health benefits[30] which are believed in part to be due to its high content of dietary fibre.[31] It is important to note that the relative proportion of dietary fibre to total carbohydrate is higher in finger millet than in other cereals, making it an ideal grain for healthy living.[32] The health benefits associated with foods rich in dietary fibre include delayed nutrient absorption, increased fecal (stool) bulk and transit time, lowering of blood lipid, and potential prevention of colon cancer.[33]

Jowar, or sorghum, is another good source of nutrients and bioactive compounds.[34] Sorghum is rich in starch, and thus is more slowly digested than other cereals.[35] It also has low digestibility proteins, unsaturated lipids, vitamins, and minerals.[36] Jowar ki roti is a type of roti/chapatti that is a healthy alternative to chapatti from processed grains. The health benefits of a multigrain diet have been shown in the laboratory in a study of adult albino female rats—one group which was fed a formulated multigrain diet (composed of millets and cereals, specifically bajra, ragi, jowar, oats, rice, and maize), and the other a commercial diet for a 10-week period. The researchers found that animals fed the multigrain diet had better health effects, including lowering of cholesterol and generating higher levels of antioxidant enzymes.[37] These findings can be translated to our diet and stresses the importance of increasing the consumption of whole, traditional grains.

In an Indian study, Shukla and colleagues compared the glycaemic index of pearl millet (bajra), barley, and corn to white bread in 18 healthy volunteers and 14 patients with type 2 diabetes. They found that glycaemic response to pearl millet and barley was significantly lower than glycaemic response to white bread, particularly in individuals who did not already have type 2 diabetes.[38]

In spite of the evidence, the regular use of these grains is spotty at best, with the perception of these grains having shifted over the decades. Whole grains have been linked to socio-economic status, with brown rice being perceived as a food of the poor and those who live in rural areas whereas the highly polished, dehusked white rice is regarded as a food of the well-off.

Kumar and colleagues conducted qualitative studies in 2009 to identify factors that were barriers to the consumption of brown rice and ways to promote its inclusion as a staple food among South Indian adults. Sixty-five adults from Chennai were split into eight focus groups and were audiotaped talking about culture and dietary practices, factors influencing rice preferences, awareness about and perceptions of brown rice, and barriers to and factors influencing acceptance of brown rice. Interestingly, participants found rice that was not white or long grained to be inferior. Some of the comments were truly telling of the challenges facing whole grains: 'If we buy this kind of rice (referring to the unmilled variety), it is a prestige issue. People will think poorly of us, it is a question of status' and 'Only if the rice is white in colour will we be satisfied and only then will our family members like to eat it…. There have been several occasions when we have bought rice from our village which was not the white variety. Our family members did eat it but they did not relish it and so I cannot cook it on a daily basis.'[39]

It is truly time to change perceptions, decrease the consumption of refined grains and head back in time to our roots, and make the nutrient-rich ancient whole grains sexy again. Following is a list of the fibre content of commonly used grains in the Indian diet to help you make good choices.

Nutrition Content of Indian Grains
(per 100 gm edible portion)

GRAINS	PROTEIN (GM)	DIETARY FIBRE (GM)	CARBOHYDRATES (GM)
• Amaranth seed, pale brown (Amaranthus cruentus)	13.27±0.34	7.47±0.09	61.46±0.60
• Bajra (Pennisetum typhoideum)	10.96±0.26	11.49±0.62	61.78±0.85
• Barley (Hordeum vulgare)	10.94±0.51	15.64±0.64	61.29±0.77
• Jowar (Sorghum vulgare)	9.97±0.43	10.22±0.49	67.68±1.03
• Maize, dry (Zea mays)	8.80±0.49	12.24±0.93	64.77±1.58
• Ragi (Eleusine coracana)	7.16±0.63	11.18±1.14	66.82±0.73
• Rice, raw, brown (Oryza sativa)	9.16±0.75	4.43±0.54	74.80±0.85
• Rice, raw, milled (Oryza sativa)	7.94±0.58	2.81±0.42	78.24±1.07
• Wheat flour, refined (Triticum aestivum)	10.36±0.29	2.76±0.29	74.27±0.92

GRAINS	PROTEIN (GM)	DIETARY FIBRE (GM)	CARBOHYDRATES (GM)
• Wheat, whole (Triticum aestivum)	10.57±0.37	11.23±0.77	64.72±1.74
• Quinoa (Chenopodium quinoa)	13.11	14.66	53.65

Source: Longvah, T. et al., *Indian Food Composition Tables 2017*, Hyderabad: National Institute of Nutrition, 2017.

An Apple a Day: The Importance of Fruits and Vegetables

Fruits and vegetables are an integral part of the Indian diet and contain compounds with numerous health benefits. The mango finds mention in the text *Shatapatha Brahmana*, which dates back to 1000 BC. Vegetables like the lotus stem (visa) and cucumber (urvaruka) find a mention in the *Rigveda*.[40] Fruits and vegetables are a very important part of a healthy, nutritious diet and are an excellent source of many vitamins and minerals, as well as dietary fibre, and can help you maintain a healthy weight as they are relatively low in calories. They have individual phytochemicals (plant-derived chemicals) that have been shown to potentially have positive effects on health. A systematic review and meta-analysis of 82 publications examined dietary risk factors for bladder cancer and found that cruciferous vegetables and citrus fruits such as oranges, lemons, lime, and grapefruit, and skim milk and fermented milk, had a protective effect and reduced the risk of bladder cancer.[41] D. Aune and colleagues published a comprehensive meta-analysis of 142 articles published between 1966 and 2016 of prospective studies examining associations between fruit and vegetable intakes and cancer, cardiovascular disease, and all-cause mortality. For fruits and vegetables combined, the lowest risk was observed at an intake of 550–600g/day (7–7.5 servings/day) for total cancer, whereas for coronary heart disease, stroke and cardiovascular disease, the lowest risk was observed at 800g/day (10 servings/day). Interestingly, of specific types of vegetables, the greatest reduction in risk in cancer was associated with green-yellow vegetables and cruciferous vegetables (cauliflower, cabbage, kale, etc.) The authors concluded 'These results support public health recommendations to increase fruit and vegetable intake for the prevention of cardiovascular disease, cancer, and premature mortality.'[42]

The European Prospective Investigation into Cancer and Nutrition (EPIC) study is a prospective cohort that includes more than 5,00,000 participants from ten European countries. When they looked at their data set they concluded that increased fruit consumption was associated with decreased cancers of the upper aerodigestive tract, such as the mouth, pharynx, larynx, and oesophagus.[43] This risk reduction was modest and the benefit was not seen for vegetable consumption. The risk of colorectal cancer was also decreased with increased intake of total fruit and vegetables and total fibre. Apart from a direct reduction in risk, daily fruit intake can decrease obesity and have an indirect effect on decreasing the risk of developing cancer. The American Cancer Society recommends eating at least 2.5 cups of fruit every day as part of the daily diet. The Expert Committee of the Indian Council of Medical Research recommends at least 300 gm of vegetables and 100 gm of fresh fruits daily.[44]

Fibre Is Our Friend

There are many health benefits associated with foods rich in dietary fibre, which include delayed nutrient absorption, decreasing the glycaemic index, increased fecal (stool) bulk, lowering of blood lipids, and increased fecal transit time.[45] Dietary fibre has been hypothesized to decrease the risk of colorectal cancer by leading to increased stool bulk and dilution of carcinogens in the colonic lumen and reduced transit time.[46] A systemic review and meta-analyses found that a high intake of dietary fibre, in particular cereal fibre and whole grains, was associated with a reduced risk of colorectal cancer.[47] In addition, findings from EPIC found that persons with higher total dietary fibre intakes had lower risk of developing colorectal or liver cancer.[48]

A study funded in part by the World Health Organization, published in *The Lancet*, reviewed 185 prospective studies and 58 clinical trials with 4,635 adult participants to establish an evidence base for quantitative recommendations for intakes of dietary fibre. The results of the study published in 2019 concluded that observational data suggested a 15–30 per cent decrease in all-cause and cardiovascular related mortality, and incidence of coronary heart disease, stroke, type 2 diabetes, and colorectal cancer when comparing the highest dietary fibre consumers with the lowest consumers. The clinical trials showed significantly lower body weight, systolic blood pressure, and total cholesterol when comparing higher with lower intakes of dietary fibre. The best outcomes were achieved when daily intake of dietary fibre was between 25 gm and 29 gm. There was a suggestion that higher intakes of dietary fibre could even protect against cardiovascular diseases, type 2 diabetes, and colorectal and breast cancers. All this points to one conclusion: fibre is most definitively our friend.[49]

...Not That

Limiting Red Meat and Processed Meats

The market for processed meat is rising rapidly in India which, according to recent surveys, is one of the fastest growing markets for processed meat and poultry globally. This increase is possibly attributed to evolving eating habits, marked by a shift towards more snacking and the need for convenience. People, busy with their lives and jobs, are pressed for time and find it convenient to gravitate towards easily microwavable, ready-to-eat frozen foods.[50]

The International Agency for Research on Cancer (IARC), the cancer agency for the World Health Organization, in 2015 released a report of 22 experts from 10 countries who had reviewed more than 800 studies on cancer in humans in the context of intake of red meat or processed meats. They concluded that eating 50 gms of processed meat (approximately one hot dog) every day increased the relative risk of colorectal cancer by 18 per cent. They defined processed meats as meat that has been transformed through salting, curing, fermentation, smoking, or other processes to enhance flavour or improve preservation. They also found limited association of eating red meat (beef, pork, mutton, lamb) with colorectal cancer and, to a lesser extent, with pancreatic cancer and prostate cancer.[51] One of the potential causes of the association could be attributed to the food being in direct contact with a flame or a hot surface that can produce more of cancer causing chemicals such as heterocyclic amines (HCAs) and polycyclic aromatic hydrocarbons (PAHs).[52] Some of these chemicals can also form during meat processing. Cancer-causing chemicals that form during meat processing include N-nitroso compounds and PAHs.

An interesting study published in 2019 aimed to take a closer look at the association of low intakes of red and processed meat with heart disease and cancer compared to those who did not eat meat at all. This study was part of the Adventist Health Study-2 (AHS-2), a prospective cohort study of approximately 96,000 Seventh-day Adventist men and women in the United States and Canada. This was an interesting study as Adventists are a very unique population where approximately 50 per cent are vegetarians, and the rest who do consume meat do so at a very low level. This research helped in understanding the effect of low levels of red and processed meat intake compared to zero-intake in a large setting. The study also evaluated the deaths of over 7,900 individuals over an 11-year period. Of those individuals who consumed meat, 90 per cent of them only ate about two ounces or less of red meat per day. The study found that the total intake of red and processed meat was associated with relatively higher risks of deaths due to total and cardiovascular diseases, and is one of the first studies to demonstrate that eating red and processed meats, even in small amounts, may increase the risk of death from all causes, especially heart disease.[53]

The World Cancer Research Fund (WCRF) guidelines for cancer prevention suggest limiting intake of red meat (lamb, goat, pork) to less than 500 gm (18 oz.) per week, and completely avoiding or limiting to very small amounts processed meat (i.e. smoked, cured or salted, or chemically preserved meats such as hot dogs and sausages).

Sugar: The Threat Hiding in Plain Sight

In Michael Moss's book, *Salt, Sugar and Fat: How the Food Giants Hooked Us*, the Pulitzer-winning journalist investigated the inner workings of an industry that worked 24/7 to shape what people eat and capitalized on how eating habits have changed over decades.[54] It is an amazing deep dive into the painstaking research the food industry conducted to 'perfectly engineer' food that we not only like but also crave and keep coming back for more. They would hire people like Howard Moskowitz, trained in high math at Queens College and experimental psychology at Harvard, to help 'engineer' food. For example, he walked the author through his recent creation of a new soda flavour for Dr Pepper. Howard started with 59 variations of sweetness, each one slightly different than the next, subjected those to 3,000 taste tests around the country, did his high math regression analysis, fed the data into a computer and figured out which one from all the variations had the perfect amount of sweetness—not too little, not too much, just like the pudding Goldilocks ate. Howard also coined the term 'Bliss Point'—it is the perfect amount of sweetness that makes the food seem irresistible and makes our brains respond with a 'reward' [we *like* it, it tastes *good*]. The reward centre of the brain gives us a little jolt of endorphins and makes our brain remember what we did to get that reward, making us want to do it again. This part of the brain is run by the neurotransmitter dopamine.[55] Have you ever wondered why it is so hard to put that bar of chocolate down after the first bite? Yes, you've reached the 'Bliss Point'.

Sweets have traditionally been a part of the Indian diet, usually consumed after meals. This tradition has been alive since the time of the Vedas when guests were welcome to the house with madhuparka made of honey, curd, and ghee.[56] The misconception is that traditional sweets, be it candy or Indian sweets, are the only sugar containing foods in diets and if one does not indulge in desserts, then one must be cutting down one's sugar consumption drastically. Alarmingly, per capita consumption of sugar in India has risen from 22 gm/day in 2000 to 55.3 gm/day in 2010.[57] One of the biggest challenges is with the consumption of sugar sweetened beverages (such as cola) that has increased by 13 per cent per year since 1998, rising from less than 2 litres per capita to 11 litres per capita per year by 2014. Easy availability of these beverages in rural and urban areas significantly contributes to higher per capita consumption.[58] An average Indian consumes about 10 spoons of sugar a day, resulting in consumption of almost 18 kg of sugar per year.[59] However, the real issue is all of us are consuming considerable amounts of sugar in hidden forms from different processed food items: sugars that are hiding in plain sight (see Table 2). For example; did you know that ONE can of cola can have up to 40 gms of sugar, which roughly equates to 10 teaspoons of sugar? Orange juice, which has long been touted as 'healthy', can have as much as six teaspoons of sugar in a 240 ml glass.

So, STOP, THINK, and #ReadTheLabel, that is, the small print at the back of the drink can and the snack packaging that calls sugars 'energy' and can be misleading.

It is imperative to closely track all sources of sugar intake as a diet rich in sugary foods may increase risk for cancer by increasing caloric intake, insulin production, oxidative stress, and promoting weight gain and obesity.[60] Also, sugar sweetened beverages may raise insulin and glucose levels and thereby risk for obesity and diabetes which in turn are risk factors for pancreatic cancer.[61] The WCRF guidelines for cancer prevention suggest avoiding consumption of beverages with added sugar.[62]

Again, the suggestion is not to completely eliminate sweets from your diet, but instead, to eat sweets sparingly and on special and festive occasions. You may even savour it more.

Ten Foods That Are Sneaking Sugar Into Your Daily Life

FOOD/BEVERAGE	GRAMS OF SUGAR	TEASPOONS OF SUGAR
• Breakfast Cereal - one cup	Upto 20	5
• Orange Juice - 200 ml	16	4
• Ketchup - one tablespoon	4	1
• Colas	40	10
• Digestive Biscuits - 250 gm	52	13
• Chocolate Milk - 230 ml	8	2
• Flavoured Yoghurt	Upto 32	8
• Sports Drinks - 570 ml	32	8
• Granola Bars	Upto 12	3
• Energy Drinks - 240 ml	25	6

The Dark Side of the Boom: The Rise of the Western Diet

The WCRF suggests limiting intake of energy-dense foods (for example, processed energy-dense foods and readily available convenience foods prepared outside one's home, including potato chips, samosas, mixture, sweets, puffs, pastries, and so on).[63] These foods do little to add to the nutrition value and are a source of empty calories. As in America, the trend in urban India is towards increasing consumption of these high 'empty calorie' foods, sugar-sweetened drinks, and an increase in percentage of Indians eating out in restaurants.[64] The rise of double income households and longer workdays translate into less time for cooking and increasing reliance on foods outside of the home, which generally tend to have larger portions and are less nutritious than those prepared at home.[65] In an interesting study, Gulati and colleagues reported on the knowledge of, attitude towards and practice of nutrition, physical activity and other lifestyle habits in urban children and mothers in India. This was a cross-sectional observational study of 1,800 children aged 9–18 years and their mothers, using qualitative (focus group) and quantitative (semi-structured survey) data. Household family income, related socio-economic factors, and overweight mothers were most significantly associated with obesity in children as were the dietary consumption patterns (snacking, fast food, etc.). The most interesting findings were focus group discussion where children stated that 'home-cooked food is old fashioned'[66] highlighting the enormous challenges in perception facing India's dietary traditions.

The impact of introducing a Western diet to individuals who had not been exposed to it before was studied by O'Keefe and colleagues and reported in the journal *Nature Communication*.[67] They studied colon cancer, which is a disease that is more common in Western countries. Interestingly, Americans of African descent have one of the highest incidences of colon cancer in the world (65:1,00,000) as compared to rural Africans, where the incidence is one of the lowest (5:1,00,000). They employed a unique design where 20 healthy African Americans in the United States and 20 rural Africans (in South Africa from the rural Kwazulu region) were studied—first for two weeks eating their usual food, after which they were fed the intervention diet for two weeks. The Americans were given 'African style' foods (high-fibre, low-fat consisting of Hi-Maize, corn fritters, spinach, red pepper, onions, okra, tomatoes), increasing their average fibre intake from 14 to 55 gm per day and reducing their fat from 35 per cent to 16 per cent of total calories, whereas Africans were given a 'Western-style' diet (high-fat and low-fibre, consisting of foods like pancakes, hamburgers, French fries, macaroni and cheese, rice krispies, meat loaf, hash browns), reducing their fibre from 66 to 12 gm per day and increasing their fat from 16 per cent to 52 per cent.

The African Americans were housed at the University of Pittsburgh Clinical Translational Research Center, and the rural Africans were housed in a rural lodging facility, close to their homes, with full kitchen facilities. They collected stool samples and performed colonoscopies on subjects to evaluate changes in their colonic mucosa. Although the diet change was brief, both groups saw changes in their microbiomes (the trillions of bacteria that live in our gut) with the American group exhibiting a decrease in colonic mucosal inflammation and turnover of cells of the intestinal lining, and the African group exhibiting the reverse. In particular, African Americans experienced an increase in a product of fibre fermentation, butyrate, which is thought to be anti-inflammatory and plays a key role in anti-cancer pathways.

This study brings home an important point that was taught to us growing up: it is never too late to turn into a new leaf, or in this case, change one's microbiome for the better. According to Dr O'Keefe: 'In just two weeks, a change in diet from a Westernized composition to a traditional African high-fibre, low-fat diet reduced these biomarkers of cancer risk, indicating that it is likely never too late to modify the risk of colon cancer.'[68]

Alcohol: Time to Bring it Down a Peg

A common question I'm asked at parties: 'What Scotch do you like?' When I politely let the host or hostess know that I don't drink whisky, a quizzical look is followed by the question: 'But … I thought you told me that you are from Delhi?' What can I say? With due apologies to my fellow Delhiites, we are a walking cliché! Though in defence of my hosts: statistics are on their side. India consumed 1.548 billion litres of whisky in 2014, dwarfing the number two country, America, which consumed a measly 462 million litres.[69] That roughly amounts to half of the world consumption of whisky! Other than this favoured class of alcohol, in India, there is a troubling overall increase in alcohol consumption over the last few decades. The Paris-based Organization for Economic Cooperation and Development (OECD) published a report examining the economic and health implications of alcohol use. India was ranked third among a list of 40 nations, for a steep increase in alcohol intake between 1992 and 2012 (up 55 per cent over 20 years). In another study published in *The Lancet*, between 2010 and 2017, alcohol consumption in India increased by 38 per cent, from 4.3 to 5.9 litres per adult per year, whereas in Europe, consumption reduced by 12 per cent (from 11.2 to 9.8 litres). The intake is growing in low- and middle-income countries, while the total volume of alcohol consumed in high-income countries has remained stable. The authors estimate that by 2030 half of all adults will drink alcohol, and almost a quarter (23 per cent) will binge drink (defined as consuming 60 gm or more pure alcohol in one sitting once or more within 30 days). This is particularly alarming for the future as the trend of heavy drinking is increasing among the youth of the country.[70]

Figure 7: Alcohol can cause seven types of cancer

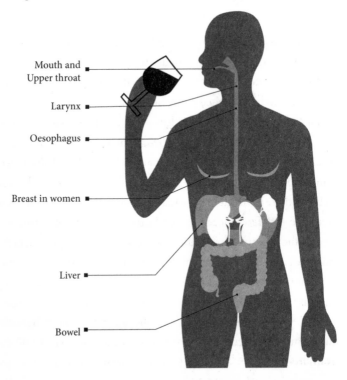

- Mouth and Upper throat
- Larynx
- Oesophagus
- Breast in women
- Liver
- Bowel

Alcohol intake, even at levels of low or moderate intake, has been associated with an increased risk of cancers of the oral cavity, pharynx, larynx, esophagus, liver, colorectum, and breast, and the risk of cancer increases as the amount of alcohol consumed increases.[71] (**Figure 7**) A recent comprehensive statistical analysis in *The Lancet* from the Global Burden of Disease Study 2016 reported that for populations aged 50 years and older, cancers accounted for a large proportion of total alcohol-attributable deaths, constituting 27.1 per cent of total female deaths and 18.9 per cent of male deaths in 2016. The authors concluded that 'Alcohol use is a leading risk factor for global disease burden and causes substantial health loss. We found that the risk of all-cause mortality, and of cancers specifically, rises with increasing levels of consumption, and the level of consumption that minimizes health loss is zero.'[72]

Along with the obvious, there are other hidden risks that lurk in the shadows. Picture this: You're with a group of friends, hanging out, discussing the latest work situation or politics of the day. A few drinks in and someone pulls out a packet of cigarettes. Maybe you smoke only occasionally and normally would have declined, but something (deep and dark inside) makes you want to reach out and grab a cigarette and light it up. You take a deep puff... and then take a few more and then drink more than you originally planned to do. Sounds familiar? Ever wonder why this happens? Scientists hypothesize that a number of factors could be at play. Central to this discussion is a neurotransmitter called dopamine which plays a major role in the reward system in our brain. The history of the discovery of the reward centre is fascinating and warrants digression.

In the 1950s, two scientists, James Olds and Peter Milner, put electrodes into the limbic system of rats' brains and sent a little shock to the area when a rat entered a particular corner.[73] They thought that the shock would be unpleasant enough to make the rats want to stay away from that corner. Instead, they noticed that when the electrodes were placed in the septal area or nucleus accumbens—one of the principal regions in which the neurotransmitter dopamine is released—the rats, rather than avoiding the corner, kept going back to get the shock over and over again, with some rats going back up 700 times within an hour! In essence, when the brain is exposed to something rewarding, it responds to the stimulus by increasing the release of dopamine: think alcohol and nicotine.

In 2013, John Dani, PhD, and his colleagues published research in *Neuron* which shed light on this connection. The study was titled 'Nicotine Decreases Ethanol-Induced Dopamine Signaling and Increases Self-Administration via Stress Hormones'. Let me explain. Alcohol and smoking independently increase the dopamine levels in the brain, increasing our happiness quotient. If you do both together, it would be safe to assume that we would feel better. But interestingly, the opposite is true. Instead of the dopamine levels going up, an increase in stress hormones made the levels go down, theoretically making us less happy. So, why do we end up drinking more? The researchers found that previous exposure to nicotine subsequently increased the tendency to drink alcohol. But then, if you smoke once you have started drinking, the level of dopamine drops, making us less happy. In order to regain that high, you have an urge to drink more and the cycle repeats.[74]

In a separate study, researchers from the University of Missouri gave rats fitted with sleep-recording electrodes alcohol and nicotine. While alcohol inhibiting the central nervous system had a depressant effect, nicotine stimulated the rat's basal forebrain, an area of the brain associated with reflexes, learning, and attention and counteracted sleepiness caused by alcohol consumption, creating a toxic nicotine-alcohol cycle.[75] Why is all of this relevant?

William Bolt and colleagues conducted a case-control study of oral (mouth) and pharyngeal (throat) cancers and their relationship to tobacco and alcohol use in 1,114 patients and 1,268 population-based controls. They found that compared with non-smokers and non-drinkers, the approximate relative risks for developing mouth and throat cancers are up to seven times greater for people who smoke tobacco and up to six times greater for those who drink alcohol. However, the risk was not additive, but almost multiplicative: a whopping **35 times greater** for those who were regular, heavy users of both substances.[76]

So, next time your friend offers you a 'Patiala Peg' (roughly 120 ml in a single serving), you may want to consider the literature and politely decline. The IARC has recommended that those who drink alcohol limit their intake and has advised that not drinking alcohol at all is better to prevent cancer.[77]

Don't 'Supplement' Real Food

Supplements to 'prevent cancer' or heal all kinds of ailments are omnipresent across the length and breadth of India. In spite of being sold as 'all natural', some of these supplements have the potential to cause real harm. The WCRF nutritional recommendations for cancer prevention discourages the use of dietary supplements for cancer prevention.[78] The enthusiasm over supplements of particular nutrients was dampened when the results of several large and highly publicized trials suggested that supplementation is not likely to be beneficial in preventing cancer, especially in well-nourished persons,[79] *and can even cause harm.*[80] For example, beta-carotene supplements have been associated with a detrimental effect on lung cancer incidence and death in persons at high-risk of lung cancer.[81] In the Alpha-Tocopherol Beta-Carotene (ATBC) study of 29,133 male smokers aged 50–69 years, beta-carotene (20 mg) increased risk of lung cancer and overall risk of dying of cancer.[82] Also, the Carotene and Retinol Efficacy Trial (CARET)—a well-designed chemoprevention trial with daily supplementation of 30 mg beta-carotene plus 25,000 IU retinyl palmitate among 18,314 heavy smokers, former heavy smokers, and asbestos-exposed workers—found that the high doses of beta-carotene and retinyl palmitate and at least one other dietary supplement increased risk of aggressive prostate cancer.[83] Furthermore, the Selenium and Vitamin E Cancer Prevention Trial (SELECT) in 35,533 healthy men found that vitamin E (400 IU/day) supplements were associated with increased risk of prostate cancer.[84]

The US Preventive Services Task Force (USPSTF) brought out recommendations for the primary prevention of cancer for the general adult population.[85] The USPSTF concluded that there is sufficient evidence to recommend *against* the use of beta-carotene or vitamin E supplements for the prevention of cancer.[86] So if you are well nourished and do not have a specific deficiency requiring supplementation, it's always better to stick to the real stuff and nourish yourself with real food.

3

Focus on the Mundane

I never thought of myself as obese. Growing up, I was the thin, scrawny, short guy who always used to stand at the front of the line in the school assembly (a phenomenon unique to the Indian subcontinent). My poor mother who was working hard to provide me with a nutritious diet was being bombarded with advice on how to 'fatten' me up and make me more 'healthy'. There were recommendations of homoeopaths in Delhi and various elixirs that promoted weight gain.

Turns out, all that worry was unwarranted as she could have just waited till I turned 30 and my metabolism slowed down. Along with the years, I had moved to the US Midwest and was working non-stop at the hospital, eating unhealthy and supersizing all my meals! Though my Body Mass Index (BMI) was approximately 25, which fell in the category of 'overweight' and not 'obese' (which was a BMI of 30 or higher), my waistline was telling me something else altogether. At first, I ignored the obvious by loosening the button on my trousers when I wore a belt, but soon it became apparent to me that the heydays of hedonistic eating without worrying about the consequences were long gone. This is an important distinction as increasingly the waist circumference or central obesity is considered to be strongly associated with an increased risk of type 2 diabetes, cardiovascular disease, and death, even if BMI is controlled. I read a lot about 'fancy' ways to get healthy (yes, I mean 'Superfoods', et al.), but in the end I settled for the *mundane:* I cut down on carbs, started working out, and tried to maintain a (mostly) healthy lifestyle!

It's Not a Diet, It's a Lifestyle Change

It's just not I who was getting 'healthy' (a 'polite' was to describe obesity in India). Using the International Obesity Task Force of the WHO (IOTF-WHO) obesity cut off of greater than 25 for Asian adults, urban India is experiencing an obesity epidemic that rivals rates in Western nations.[87] For example, in an epidemiological study (n=26,000) in Chennai, 31.2 per cent of women and 24.6 per cent of men were found to meet the IOTF-WHO definition of obesity.[88] In the New Delhi Birth Cohort Study, 54 per cent of men and 66 per cent of women were found to be obese by IOTF-WHO criteria.[89] By using a sensitive waist circumference cut off for abdominal obesity (≥80 cm in women, ≥90 cm in men) for Asian adults, 70 per cent of an epidemiological cohort in New Delhi was reported to have central obesity.[90] There also is a disturbing trend of increasing rate of obesity among Indian women, with an increase in the prevalence among reproductive-age women (15–49 years) from 9.3 per cent in 2005–06 to 20.7 per cent in 2015–16. In 25 states and Union Territories, one in every five women was obese as per the National Family Health Survey conducted in

2015–16, whereas the numbers were higher in Andhra Pradesh, Goa, Kerala, Punjab, Tamil Nadu, NCT Delhi, Chandigarh, and Puducherry, where over 30 per cent of women were obese.[91] Alarmingly, the obesity epidemic is now believed to be spreading also to the lower-income strata of adults with 50.9 per cent of low-income men and 49.8 per cent of low-income women in Chennai experiencing central obesity.[92] These temporal trends are attributed at least partially to the rapid urbanization of India.[93] However, rural India is also experiencing an emerging problem with weight and obesity.[94] Very troubling is the emergence of a 'double burden' of malnutrition and obesity in rural India.[95] This is truly worrisome as 'junk food' has penetrated into all corners of India.

Obesity can lead to altered levels of hormones like insulin, insulin-like growth factor-1, leptin, adiponectin, steroid hormones, and cytokines, which have the potential to create an environment in the body that favours cancer development and progression.[96]

Nearly all of the evidence linking obesity to cancer risk comes from large cohort studies, which is a type of observational study. A hospital based case-control study from Mumbai concluded that central obesity appears to be a key risk factor for breast cancer irrespective of menopausal or hormone receptor status in Indian women with no history of hormone replacement therapy.[97] In spite of the limitations of the study designs, there is consistent evidence that higher amounts of body fat are associated with increased risks of various cancers, as listed in the figure. (**Figure 8**)

The WCRF International recommendations for cancer prevention suggest that adults should maintain their body weight within the normal range and avoid weight gain and increases in waist circumference all through adulthood.[98]

Figure 8: Cancers Associated with Being Overweight & Obesity

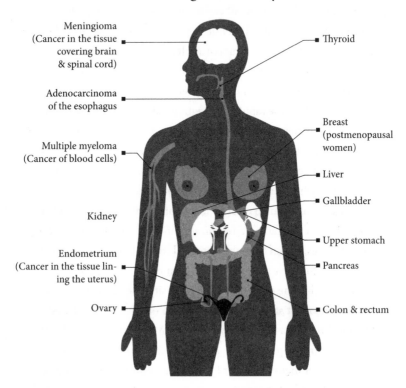

Meningioma (Cancer in the tissue covering brain & spinal cord)

Thyroid

Adenocarcinoma of the esophagus

Breast (postmenopausal women)

Multiple myeloma (Cancer of blood cells)

Liver

Gallbladder

Kidney

Upper stomach

Endometrium (Cancer in the tissue lining the uterus)

Pancreas

Ovary

Colon & rectum

Exercise: The Body Achieves What the Mind Believes

Exercise—the brief thought that creeps into our minds around the New Year and has fled away by February. I know it's hard, but regular physical activity does have many benefits, including reducing your risk of certain cancers. A meta-analysis of 52 epidemiologic studies examined the association between physical activity and the risk of developing colon cancer and found that the individuals who were most physically active had a 24 per cent lower risk of colon cancer than those who were the least physically active.[99] Similar findings have been noted with breast cancer, where physical activity has been associated with a reduced risk of breast cancer in both premenopausal and postmenopausal women; however, the evidence is stronger for women who are postmenopausal. It may also be beneficial to increase your physical activity after menopause as women who do so may have a lower risk of breast cancer than women who do not.[100]

So how much should we exercise? Exercise intensity is often defined in terms of METs, or metabolic equivalents. One MET is the amount of energy it takes to sit quietly. Moderate-intensity activities are activities that get one moving fast enough or strenuously enough to burn off three to six times as much energy per minute as one does while sitting quietly; in other words, exercises that burn three to six METs. Examples of moderate intensity activity include brisk walking and doubles tennis. Vigorous-intensity activities burn over six METs.[101] Examples of vigorous intensity activity include singles tennis, race walking, jogging or running, swimming laps, aerobic dancing, bicycling (10 miles per hour or faster), jumping rope or heavy gardening (for example, continuous digging). Several internationally recognized guidelines for physical activity recommend weekly 150 minutes of moderate-intensity activity, 75 minutes of vigorous-intensity activity, or a combination of moderate and vigorous activity with two days of resistance training.[102] Though strong evidence is still accruing, exercise and weight control have been offered as opportunities to reduce risk of developing multiple different cancers, including prostate cancer.[103]

The WCRF International recommendations for cancer suggest a minimum moderate physical activity, such as brisk walking, for at least 30 minutes each day, and limiting sedentary practices such as watching television.[104] The WCRF further recommends that the ideal would be more than 60 minutes of moderate, or more than 30 minutes vigorous physical activity each day.[105] A large study from the Indian Council of Medical Research was conducted in four regions of India (Tamil Nadu, Maharashtra, Jharkhand, and Chandigarh) which represented south, west, east and north of India respectively. These areas had a combined population of 213 million people. Physical activity was assessed using the Global Physical Activity Questionnaire (GPAQ) in 14,227 individuals aged 20 years and above, both in urban (4,173) and in rural (10,054) areas. Shockingly, a majority (54.4 per cent) were inactive, with only 13 per cent being highly active. The inactivity was more in urban areas (65 per cent)as compared to rural areas (50 per cent). People spent the majority of their time at work with a near absence of recreational physical activity, as reported by a whopping 88.4, 94.8, 91.3 and 93.1 per cent of the subjects in Chandigarh, Jharkhand, Maharashtra, and Tamil Nadu respectively. [106]

There is an urgent need to promote recreational physical activity in India. Remember: the hardest part of a workout is to get your body off that couch! So, don't let that treadmill be a stand for drying clothes. It is time to get off that couch, turn off the television, and keep your phone away. GET moving and GET fit: Bhaag India bhaag!

Breastfeeding

Breastfeeding has been associated with a reduced risk of breast cancer in both premenopausal and postmenopausal women.[107]

In a study by the Collaborative Group on Hormonal Factors in Breast Cancer, researchers found that for every 12 months a woman breastfed, her relative risk of breast cancer decreased by 4.3 per cent in addition to a decrease in 7 per cent for each birth. Breastfeeding also exerts a modest protective effect against endometrial and ovarian cancers.[108] In a population of Chinese women, it was found that women who breastfed for more than 13 months were 63 per cent less likely to develop ovarian cancer than women who breastfed for less than seven months. Women who breastfed multiple children for more than 31 months could reduce their ovarian cancer risk by up to 91 per cent as compared to women who breastfed for less than 10 months.

The hypothesis is that women who breastfeed have fewer menstrual cycles throughout their lives, and therefore less exposure to estrogen, which can promote breast cancer growth. Similarly, breastfeeding can potentially help lower the risk of ovarian cancer, preventing ovulation, and leading to reduced exposure to estrogen.

Here exists a silver lining: the percentage of infants (under six months of age) who were exclusively breastfed in India increased from 46.4 per cent to 54.9 per cent from 2006 to 2016. There was, however, variability in the data with the prevalence of exclusive breastfeeding ranging from 35.8 per cent in Meghalaya to 77.2 per cent in Chhattisgarh. Despite this variability in levels, most states saw substantial increases in rates of exclusive breastfeeding.[109]

4

Prevention Is the Cure

My parents told me this when I was growing up and I tell my kids now: There are no easy fixes or shortcuts in life. This is especially true when it comes to your overall health. India is an amazing land of diverse peoples and cultures with palates and dietary preferences that are even more varied. The last two decades delivered an economic boom with rapid urbanization, leading to an increase in disposable income and heralding a sea change in dietary and lifestyle habits, seriously impacting overall health and well-being.

The 'good' news is that traditional Indian diets already did incorporate elements that the ACS recommends: a plant-based diet that is fibre rich. Dietary fibre has been linked to a lower risk of some types of cancer, especially colorectal cancer. The 'bad' part is that the Indian diet is also overrun with food and snacks that are low in fibre and high in carbohydrate and fat: our samosas, sweets (jalebi, halwa), bhaturas, naans, parathas, just to name a few. The 'ugly' part is that over the past few decades, processed food has become a staple in the Indian diet. This is a cause of great concern for our children's health. TV, billboards, and the internet have inundated our households with ads for calorie bombs like pizza, fries, and sugary drinks. This, along with a sedentary lifestyle, is a recipe for disaster.

Expert Recommendations

Nutritional recommendations for cancer prevention have been formulated by the WCRF and the ACS.[110] The WCRF International recommendations for cancer prevention include maintaining healthy body weight and avoiding weight gain and increases in waist circumference throughout adulthood; limiting the intake of energy-dense foods (foods that have a lot of calories relative to nutrients) such as fried foods and foods with added sugar (desserts and sweets); eating mostly plant-based foods; and most importantly, meeting one's nutritional needs from diet alone rather than using dietary supplements to protect against cancer.[111]

The ACS recommends that one should 'choose foods and drinks in amounts that help you get to and maintain a healthy weight, limit how much processed meat and red meat you eat, eat at least two and a half cups of vegetables and fruits each day and choose whole grains instead of refined grain products'.[112]

Get Started Yesterday

If you've read this far, it means you are committed to starting your overall health and nutrition journey. Trying to improve your health is not like a 100-metre dash, it is more akin to running a marathon with hurdles. And if you slow down, you can use these hashtags to help keep you motivated and on track:

#FitnessBuddy

On my way to work, I used to drive by gyms and always thought that one day I would enter and start working out. That never happened. Then came the treadmill that was parked in a room in our house—I think my kids played on it more than anyone ever using it for exercise. Finally, I decided to pay for that gym membership, my reasoning being that if you pay for something you are more likely to use it, right? Wrong again: that was a spectacular failure! The first month I did venture in for a few days, but then there was always an excuse: life is so busy, work is crazy, yada yada.

After 'window shopping' for over a decade, I finally started on my wellness journey. What helped me was the fitness community that was around me, including my friends, and most of all, my #FitnessBuddy: my wife! The moral of the story is that you do not have to do this alone: there are always people to help you out. It makes achieving your health goals a lot more fun. Beginning a health regimen is always hard and requires a lot of motivation. Having a 'health' or 'fitness' family who can continue to encourage you can help make this transition easier.

#ReliableSources

In this day and age of 'fake news', it is imperative to verify sources and not to mindlessly share a sensational story on social media about cancer without doing your own research, as sharing misinformation can result in real world consequences. It is also important to not dismiss stories just because they are not aligned with your world view: Be open-minded, venture out of your echo chamber. Be agnostic: follow the data and not unreliable opinions.

#KFS

Life is complicated, so #KeepFoodSimple. Diet 'fads' are just that: objects or behaviours that achieve short-lived popularity but fade away. Be consistent. Focus on the mundane and not just the new 'sexy' diet trend in town. Don't get stuck on single food groups: find the right balance of protein, carbohydrates, fats, and minerals. Variety, as they say, is truly the spice of life when it comes to food.

#DineIn

With the rise of disposable incomes and double income households, it is now increasingly common to dine out. This can contribute to obesity as it is well known that when food is prepared at home, it normally has less calories, sugars, and fats and is more nutritious than food in restaurants.[113] Home-cooked food also has a bad name, with children labelling it as 'old-fashioned'. Take a calendar and make a list of how many times you ate out in the last month. Now, work backwards to identify how many were for special occasions and how many times could you have easily eaten at home, but chose to go out. Try and track this for the months ahead. If you eat out, be discerning of the restaurants you choose; avoid the big chains and focus on small mom-and-pop places where you can have more confidence about what they put in their food. Question the servers/managers in the restaurant to understand the ingredients and see if this agrees with your nutrition goals. And most importantly, involve your children in this gastronomic journey so that they recognize the benefits of home-cooked food.

#JustSayNo

One word for tobacco: No. This is the most important decision you can take to decrease your risk of developing cancer, along with a host of other health benefits in addition. All tobacco, not only the smoking kind, can increase your risk of cancer. If you smoke or use tobacco products, it is never too late to quit. Work with your friends, family, and physicians to get a programme in place to quit.

#MakeGrainsSexyAgain

Before the 1950s, whole grains were commonplace in India, but their use steadily dwindled down to be replaced by the more refined and processed grains. Reduce the use of refined grains, and head back in time to our roots, and experiment with traditional whole grains like jowar, ragi, and amaranth for a 'whole'some diet.

#FoodTracker

To reach a goal, we first have to understand where we stand currently. An important first step is to keep a food diary for a week and evaluate the calories you are consuming. Next, break down the food into 'healthy' (fruits, vegetables, etc.) and 'unhealthy' (sugar containing beverages, refined carbohydrates, etc.). Capture everything! (Yes, even that small snack or samosa that you had with tea). Now that you have a baseline, try and make changes towards a healthy, wholesome diet (more fruits, less red and processed meats) and you will be surprised at the outcome.

#RealFoodNotPills

Getting on a path to wellness is hard, popping a pill is easy. If you don't harbour a specific deficiency, a supplement may cause more harm than good, which is especially true for smokers. Just as you would not take medicines without expert advice, do the same for supplements. Better still, focus on a nutritious diet from food instead of gravitating towards a magic bullet in the form of a pill.

#ReadTheLabel

This is one of the most critical elements of your health journey. Before you consume anything, look at the back of the packaging in small font and you will be amazed at how many empty calories hide in plain sight. For example, did you know that a can of cola can contain as many as 10 teaspoons of sugar? So, be an informed customer. Before you buy anything, be sure to look at the back and #ReadTheLabel.

#GetUpGetOut

Though the focus is on diet, food and exercise are synergistic and they work to complement each other and improve your overall health. And for exercise, you don't have to do the P90X. Start small with a daily walk or a short run; just about anything that will get your body moving and blood pumping through your muscles.

I hope you are convinced that it is truly time to rethink our priorities. Kick-start a healthy lifestyle with a change in your diet and regular exercise. It is essential to persevere rather than succumb to a quick food fad or eating more of the so-called 'superfoods'. Remember the saying that relates to life in general and cancer in specific: If it sounds too good to be true, it probably is. If you truly want to decrease your risk, focus on the mundane, not the 'sexy' solutions: there is no substitute for weight loss, exercise, and a well-balanced, healthy diet. It's time to unleash your creative self and combine traditional grains with a modern flair to create delectable dishes. Here are a few recipes to get you started. Bon appetit!

....

TURMERIC

....

It is the ingredient used in Ayurvedic medicine as a traditional remedy for discomfort and inflammation for 5,000 years[114] and, in more contemporary times, helps add flavour to your favourite 'chai' latte. Curcumin is a bright yellow-coloured hydrophobic polyphenol found in the rhizome of turmeric (Curcuma longa).[115] It has long been believed to have various health benefits on account of its antioxidant and anti-inflammatory mechanisms, which have been proven in laboratory studies as well.[116]

However, curcumin is only slightly water-soluble, which causes tremendous difficulties when orally administered, and is not easily absorbed by the body.[117] Also, patients report poor tolerance when curcumin is administered in bulk.[118] Multiple strategies are being evaluated when it comes to increasing the absorption, including co-administering or combining with piperine (an alkaloid found in black pepper) and resveratrol (a naturally occurring compound found in red and purple grapes, blueberries, cranberries, peanuts), and trying to design nanocurcumin particles. Though curcumin has demonstrated benefits in the cells lines of mice, it is unknown if this effect occurs when given to humans. Oral curcumin has been tested in clinical trials in combination with chemotherapy, with disappointing results and a low response rate in patients. The most commonly used dose of oral curcumin has been 8 gm/day in clinical trials, with the main side effect being fullness in the belly and pain, which led to the reduction in dose for some patients.[119] Overall, turmeric has shown effectiveness in the laboratory. However, its clinical use still requires further investigation. Intake of turmeric as part of a daily diet may have long-term health benefits; however, supplementation with high dose oral curcumin has had its limitations in the prevention and treatment of cancer. Poor absorption, poor tolerance when taken in bulk, poor water solubility, rapid degradation, fast breakdown, and quick elimination limit the use of curcumin as a novel agent in cancer therapy.[120]

Recipes

CONTRIBUTED BY PUSHPESH PANT

Barley (Jau) Pulao

Serves 3–4

Preparation time: 10–15 minutes

Cooking time: 20–25 minutes

INGREDIENTS

1–1½ cups barley

1 medium onion, peeled and sliced finely

½ cup peas, shelled

3–4 cauliflower florets (medium sized)

1 medium carrot, scraped and diced

1 tsp ginger–garlic paste

1 bay leaf

2–3 cloves

1 brown cardamom

1 inch piece of cinnamon stick

½ tsp all-spice powder

½ tsp red chilly powder

¼ tsp turmeric powder

¼ tsp black peppercorn powder

½ cup butter/ghee

3–3½ cups chicken or vegetable stock

1 tsp lemon juice

2 green chillies, deseeded and slit lengthwise

A sprig of mint leaves, for garnishing

Salt to taste

INSTRUCTIONS

Heat the butter or ghee in a pan. Add onion and stir-fry till it is rich brown. Remove and place on absorbent paper to remove excess fat. Now put in the bay leaf and whole spices. When these begin to change colour, add garlic–ginger paste. Stir briskly and add the vegetables. Stir-fry for about a minute and then add the jau grains. Stir-fry for couple of minutes before pouring in the stock and powdered spices along with salt. Cook covered till all moisture is absorbed. Check once or twice in between and stir. Once it is cooked, add lemon juice. Fluff with a fork and garnish with fried onion and mint leaves.

Barley (Jau) Thukpa Stew

Serves 2
Preparation time: 20 minutes
Cooking time: 25–30 minutes

INGREDIENTS

1 cup barley flour
200 gm boneless chicken, cut into bite-sized pieces
1 medium onion, peeled and chopped
2 medium potatoes, peeled and quartered
2 medium carrots, peeled and cut into pieces
1 small bunch of spinach leaves, chopped coarsely
1 small head of cabbage, quartered and then cut into halves
1tsp red chilli powder
1tsp cumin powder (optional)
2–3 green chillies, chopped
1 inch piece of ginger, scraped and chopped
4 cups chicken or vegetable stock
½ cup oil or butter
Salt to taste

INSTRUCTIONS

Knead the jau flour with a little water until it is soft and pliable. Then, pinch out small portions of the dough to make small flat pieces, about 2 inches long. Keep this aside. Heat oil or butter in a pan, then pour the stock and add the pieces of chicken. Boil for 10 minutes and then add all the vegetables and powdered spices along with salt. Cook covered for about 15 minutes, or till the chicken and vegetables are done. Now add the dough pieces and boil over a low or medium heat. Cook for about 5 minutes. Adjust the seasoning as needed. Enjoy while it's hot.

NOTES

If you want to have a vegetarian stew, substitute the chicken with paneer or tofu chunks. You may also use both.

Sorghum (Jowar) Upma

Serves 2
Preparation time: 5 minutes
Cooking time: 25 minutes

INGREDIENTS

1 cup sorghum
1 cup assorted vegetables (tomatoes, carrots, beans/shelled peas), chopped
1 small onion, peeled and sliced finely
1 inch piece of ginger, scraped and diced small
½ tsp cumin seeds
½ tsp fenugreek seeds
½ tsp mustard seeds

1 tsp urad/chana dal

2 green chillies, deseeded and slit lengthwise

1 whole red chilli

A pinch of turmeric (optional)

2 tbsp ghee/oil

1 tsp lemon juice

A small sprig of curry leaves

1 tbsp cashew nuts, roasted

Salt to taste

INSTRUCTIONS

Clean, pick, and wash well the jowar grains several times. Soak in water overnight. Pressure cook the grains in three cups of water for three whistles. Allow the pressure to release by itself. If needed, cook uncovered to evaporate the remaining water. Heat oil in a pan and add mustard, fenugreek and cumin seeds, along with lentils and the whole red chilli and curry leaves. When the seeds splutter, add onion and green chilies. Add jowar grains and fluff with a fork. Add turmeric and salt. Mix well. Sprinkle a little water. Stir-fry vegetables for a minute in a separate pan with very little oil before adding them to the upma.

NOTES

Cook covered on low heat for a couple of minutes, adding a little water if required. Sprinkle a little lemon juice and garnish with cashew nuts before serving.

Sorghum (Jowar) Dosa

Serves 2
Preparation time: 5 minutes
Cooking time: 25 minutes

INGREDIENTS

½ cup sorghum
½ cup rice
½ cup urad dal, husked
1 tbsp methi (fenugreek) seeds
Ghee/oil, to pan-grill

INSTRUCTIONS

Soak jowar grains in water overnight. Soak the rice and urad dal along with methi seeds separately for 6–8 hours. Grind jowar, rice, and urad dal with methi to a medium-thick batter, mixing in a sufficient amount of water. Then, mix both together. Blend this dosa batter well to a smooth batter of dropping consistency and store in a cool place to ferment for 6–8 hours. Lightly grease a pan (spread a very thin film of oil or ghee if using a non-stick pan) and pour a ladle of dosa batter. Spread in a circular motion to cover the pan's surface. Sprinkle a few drops of ghee or oil along the edges. Gently flip over when the dosa is browned at the edges and blisters bubble up all over. Cook on medium or low heat for a minute and fold into a half-moon or crescent.

Pearl Millet (Bajra) Thalipeeth

Serves 2
Preparation time: 5 minutes
Cooking time: 30 minutes

INGREDIENTS

100 gm bajra flour
100 gm ragi (finger millet flour)
2 tbsp rice flour
1 medium onion, chopped
Green chillies, chopped, as per taste
½ tbsp garlic paste
½ tbsp ajwain
Oil, as required
Warm water, for kneading
Salt to taste

INSTRUCTIONS

Mix all the ingredients together by adding warm water and knead into a dough. Make small balls of the dough. Apply some oil on a plastic sheet and press each ball into a flat circle. Create a hole in the centre. Shallow fry in a pan. Remove from the flame and place them on a paper napkin. Serve hot with chutney, tomato sauce or pickle.

Amaranth with Green Vegetables
(Chaulai ka Saag)

Serves 4–6

Preparation time: 7–8 minutes

Cooking time: 15–20 minutes

INGREDIENTS

1–2 kg chaulai leaves

2–3 whole red chillies

1 tbsp cumin seeds

2–3 garlic cloves, crushed

A pinch of asafoetida

2 tbsp vegetable oil

Salt to taste

INSTRUCTIONS

Wash the chaulai and chop finely. Heat oil in a deep pan. Add the red chillies and cumin seeds. Add garlic cloves and asafoetida. Then add the greens and salt. Cover and simmer for 10–12 minutes. Let the water dry. Serve it with bread.

Amaranth Sweet
(Chaulai ke Laddoo)

Serves 6–8

Preparation time: 10–15 minutes

INGREDIENTS

500 gm chaulai

250 gm sugar

Cardamom, for flavouring

INSTRUCTIONS

Roast the chaulai lightly. Prepare sugar syrup by dissolving sugar in water and boiling till the syrup is sticky. Add enough quantity of the syrup to the chaulai to be able to roll small balls. Give final touches to the laddoos by rolling them on powdered cardamom. Honey could also be used to sweeten the laddoos. Place the balls to dry on a lightly greased plate.

Finger Millet (Ragi) Onion Chapatti

Serves 2
Preparation time: 5 minutes
Cooking time: 30 minutes

INGREDIENTS

100 gm ragi flour
1 medium onion, chopped
2–3 green chillies
Yoghurt, as required
Coriander leaves, as required
Oil, as required
Salt to taste

INSTRUCTIONS

Add all the ingredients and knead them into a soft dough. Now heat a pan and grease it with oil. Make equal-sized balls of the dough and make them into small rotis with hand by applying a little oil to your palms. Transfer the roti to the pan and cook it on a low flame. Once done, flip it over the other side. Now serve it with yoghurt, pickle or any curry.

Pearl Millet (Bajra) Khichdi

Serves 2

Preparation time: 5 minutes

Cooking time: 25 minutes

INGREDIENTS

2 cups whole bajra, soaked overnight

1 cup whole moong dal, soaked overnight

5 peppercorns

3–4 cloves

1 tbsp cumin seeds

A pinch of asafoetida

¼ tsp turmeric powder

1 tbsp ghee

5 cups water

INSTRUCTIONS

Grind the bajra coarsely. Wash the dal. Heat ghee in a pan and add peppercorn, cloves, and cumin seeds. When the cumin seeds crackle, add asafoetida, turmeric, salt, dal, bajra, and five cups of water. Cook on medium flame. Stir when the mixture begins to boil. Cook until the bajra is soft. Add more water to get the preferred consistency. Serve hot with ghee or yoghurt, pickles, and papad.

Eating Healthy During Cancer Therapy

Float like a butterfly, sting like a bee.

—MUHAMMAD ALI

Muhammad Ali is widely regarded as one of the greatest boxers of all times. He was just 22 years old when he won the world heavyweight championship from Sonny Liston in a major upset. Ali was legendary for his clean, healthy eating habits and his dedication to his gruelling training routine. When patients ask me about what to eat while undergoing therapy, I often liken it to training for a championship bout. Just like championship fighters always watch what they eat and prep for the championship, similarly, patients fighting cancer need to dedicate time and energy into what to eat during cancer therapy as it places a lot of nutritional demands on the body.

Though the stories in this book are of women who have undergone therapy for breast cancer, the concepts of what to eat during cancer therapy is widely applicable to BOTH men and women and to other cancers including, but not limited to, prostate, ovarian, and lung cancer. In addition, it is important to remember that everyone's situation can be different based on geography, economic status, body habitus, eating habits, etc.

There are also special situations like patients with head and neck cancer who cannot eat well on account of surgery or radiation. They may require additional nutritional support with external tube feeds or intravenously, through a process called Total Parenteral Nutrition(TPN), in order to maintain their nutritional status. Another example is in patients with cancer of the pancreas, who have a tough time breaking down fats and maintaining their lean muscle mass. They frequently require supplementation with pancreatic enzymes given in the form of pills.

The suggestions in this book are based on existing scientific knowledge but are not intended to be medical advice or to replace advice by your physicians. It is important to address any medical questions to your healthcare team. Try and stay hydrated during your treatments. Practice good mouth care by brushing your tongue and teeth after each meal. You can try baking soda rinse to cleanse your palette. Wash fruits and vegetables well and cook food to proper temperatures. Gather your support group around, write down what sounds good, and make a meal plan for the day and week ahead. Cancer therapy can be a long, drawn-out fight and it is of utmost importance to stay healthy and nourished throughout the process. Channel your inner Ali, put your cancer-fighting gloves on, and get ready to fight cancer. Don't worry, you are not in this alone. At the end of this section, we have included recipes from chefs and cancer survivors to help you on your journey. Bon appetit, Cancer Warriors!

1

Managing Your Nutritional Needs

Anjali Sapra was in shock. The doctor was speaking, but she was finding it difficult to comprehend what was being said. Breast cancer again? How? This was déjà vu at its worst. Only two years ago, she was enjoying a happy, contented life as a wife, mother, and celebrated artist with shows in India and abroad before it had all come crashing down in a heartbeat.

It was close to the end of December, when she was changing one night, that she felt something different: there was a lump in her right breast that she did not remember feeling before. The thought of cancer never crossed her mind as she considered herself healthy and had no case of cancer in the family. However, to be certain that there was nothing wrong, she went to her gynaecologist on 30 December and received the dreaded diagnosis of cancer on New Year's Eve. This news was devastating and she felt she was stuck in a nightmare. Advice poured in from all directions: friends, family members, doctors. The vibes were overwhelmingly positive, though some were decidedly unhelpful ('This is karma'). She felt numb with an overload of information, all of which was alien to her.

Anxiety and thoughts of mortality set in. Things moved quickly, and less than a month after her diagnosis and surgery, she began chemotherapy. Her body reacted almost instantly and she was admitted to the hospital with infection due to a low white count manifesting as rapidly increasing high fever and body aches. While she recovered after 10 days, her taste buds changed: the sensation of salt remained, but sugary food (especially chocolate, which she loved) now tasted like soap and smells of cooking were now unpleasant.

Though Anjali's struggles after the initial round of chemotherapy was on account of infection, a number of patients with a cancer diagnosis can experience decreased appetite and loss of weight, even when they do not have any signs or symptoms of infection. In fact, for many cancer patients, *involuntary, unintended* or *unexplained* weight loss maybe the first sign of the disease and can occur in approximately 15–40 per cent of patients at the time of diagnosis and in up to 80 per cent of patients with advanced cancer. The European Society for Clinical Nutrition and Metabolism (ESPEN) developed guidelines for nutrition in cancer patients, and indicated that malnutrition, especially, should be given attention.[121]

Patients with cancer, especially with advanced cancer, can also experience a syndrome called cancer related anorexia and cachexia. Anorexia is defined as a lack or loss of appetite for food (as a medical condition). The term cachexia has Greek origins, a combination of the words kakós (bad things) and hexus (condition or state of being). It has been recognized over centuries, with Hippocrates describing a syndrome of wasting of patients who were ill as 'the flesh is consumed and becomes water, the abdomen fills with water, the feet and legs swell, the shoulders, clavicles, chest, and thighs melt away... The illness is fatal.'[122] For cancer patients, this is defined as a 'multifactorial syndrome defined by an ongoing loss of skeletal muscle mass (with or without loss of fat mass) that cannot be fully reversed by conventional nutritional support and leads to progressive functional impairment'.[123] In cancer cachexia, there is a disproportionate loss of skeletal muscle mass (also defined as sarcopenia) as opposed to loss of adipose tissue (fat), which is already less. It is due to many factors like loss of appetite and the release of substances called 'cytokines' by the body. This decreases the production and increases the breakdown of protein and fat in a double whammy to the body. Interestingly, obese patients can also suffer from cancer-associated weight loss as, in spite of being overweight, they can often lose their lean muscle mass (sarcopenia) and can be muscle 'skinny' while their BMI is still in the obese range. Malnutrition in cancer patients is multifactorial and can occur due to insufficient food intake, ulcers in the mouth, dry mouth, diarrhoea, vomiting, reduced physical activity, and metabolic derangements (such as elevated resting metabolic rate, insulin resistance, breakdown of protein and fat which increase weight loss), and as a result of anticancer therapy.[124] There is evidence that some cancer patients may have a high Resting Energy Expenditure (REE) that is defined as the energy expenditure of a person, who is not fasting, when he or she is lying down. REE has been found to be elevated in patients with lung cancer and pancreatic cancer. Essentially, these patients are burning calories at rest! This is a problem in patients with cancer as they have a more difficult time gaining or maintaining weight. A study conducted at the All India Institute of Medical Sciences in 148 patients with advanced lung cancer found that 46.6 per cent of patients were hyper-metabolic with higher than normal resting energy expenditure, and that 31 per cent were cachexic with lower than recommended intakes of calories and proteins.[125] Although these patients were expending more energy, they were not eating more.[126]

ESPEN has formulated guidelines for nutrition in cancer patients. They indicate that all cancer patients should be screened at the time of diagnosis and regularly for malnutrition and should receive counselling for nutrition.[127] As lean muscle mass is broken down, protein intake is very important and patients should try and eat 1 to 1.5 gm of protein/kg of body weight/day. That is, if your weigh 60 kgs, your daily intake should be between 60 gms to 90 gms of protein. As protein is excreted from your body by your kidneys, you should always let your doctor know about your food intake and may have to adjust if your kidneys are not working well. Along with diet, it is important to be active and include physical therapy as a component during cancer therapy. There is strong evidence that physical activity is well-tolerated and safe at different stages of cancer and that cancer patients, even those in the advanced stages of the disease, are willing to engage in physical activity.[128] Physical exercise can include light weights to get in a component of resistance training to increase muscle mass and strength. Cancer is a catabolic process, with the body being in a constant 'breakdown' mode. Exercise helps to promote anabolism, increase muscle, and build the body back up by retaining and utilizing the nutrients in the body. You don't need to head to a gym. If exercising is not your thing, try and at least get a daily walk in to prevent the muscles from wasting.

Lack of appetite is a common issue for patients with cancer and these simple tips may help keep you healthy during cancer therapy:[129]

- Eat multiple small meals, instead of three large meals. This can prevent the feeling of being too full. Eat whatever, whenever. Eat breakfast for dinner if that is what you feel like doing.

- Keep snacks easily accessible so that they are available when you feel like eating. Carry snacks that are easy to eat when you go out. And don't forget to get in that bedtime snack. Examples of healthy snacks include fruit, nuts, yoghurt, pudding, hard-boiled eggs, and granola bars.

- Make every bite count. Try adding extra protein and calories when possible and limit foods with high fats.

- Liquids are your friend. It is important to keep a bottle nearby to drink liquids throughout the day and not be dehydrated. Again, the same concept as above applies: make each sip count by choosing liquids that add calories and nutrients like protein shakes, fat-free or low-fat milk, smoothies, and avoiding filling yourself up with non-calorie fluids, such as caffeinated beverages.

- Try new foods. Don't be afraid to experiment. Taste buds are constantly changing during cancer therapy; foods can taste too sweet or salty and it is important to listen to your body and adjust to your changing taste.

- Avoid snacks that may make any treatment-related side effects worse. If you have diarrhoea, for example, avoid high fibre foods. If you have a sore or dry mouth and throat, do not eat dry, coarse snacks and maybe try something cool and soothing. The Academy of Nutrition and Dietetics recommends that patients may find relief by eating soft and liquid foods, such as yoghurt, smoothies, eggs, pudding, mashed potatoes, or warm soup.[130] Blend your foods and try softening with milk, gravy, broth, or sauces.[131] Patients can also try frozen grapes, watermelon, or peach slices. Avoid irritating or acidic foods, such as citrus or citrus-derived foods, dry foods, hot coffee, hot tea, alcohol, and foods that have tiny seeds.[132]

- Though this was not the case with Anjali, instead of weight loss, some patients might experience weight gain and increased appetite due to stress, anxiety, cancer therapy, or hormonal changes. For these patients, weight gain can be avoided by exercising self-discipline and not resorting to eating unhealthy food as a natural response to stress or anxiety, but by making healthy food choices when snacking.[133] Examples of healthy snacks include fruit, vegetables, and yoghurt.[134] Try and engage yourself in activities that you enjoy to counter stress and anxiety.[135] Cancer hospitals and centres may offer support groups, art therapy, massages, or other coping options.[136]

Initially, things were tough for Anjali, but she adjusted with time. Yoghurt and khichdi (when dealing with mouth sores), lime and tomato became her go-to foods. To increase her protein intake, she ate lightly sautéed fish, eggs and chicken liver along with daily servings of lentils. She discovered a repertoire of soups that she relied on. She also enjoyed a glass of fresh pressed orange juice every day, coconut water and a serving of pomegranate daily. Binging on food programmes became a habit and she could almost taste the delicious recipes in her mouth as they were being cooked on TV! She tweaked them to make them more healthy and palatable to her altered taste buds and came up with a varied and interesting menu. The most challenging part was the fatigue she felt, but she did not let it dictate her life. There were some days she felt too drained to get out of bed, but she made a herculean effort, got up, bathed, wore her nicest clothes, put make-up on … and then went right back to bed! She did not let the fatigue break her spirit.

After a few gruelling months, she was done with therapy and was off to Goa to celebrate! Unfortunately, this joy was short-lived as during a routine follow-up after a year-and-a-half, she found out that she had another kind of cancer on the other breast. This time though, things were different. After the initial shock wore off, she adjusted. She had a support group of fellow survivors to fall back on and her daughters, who were now grown up and were her pillars of support.

As was the case with Anjali, the support of friends and family is invaluable. A qualitative study in women who had completed primary treatment for stage I–III of breast cancer found that the formal involvement of a support person such as a family member or a friend and participation in ongoing, community-based services to maintain perceived accountability in patients may be a particularly useful strategy for weight loss interventions targeting women with breast cancer.[137] Her second brush with chemotherapy went much smoother. She finished chemotherapy, she went off again to the sunny shores of Goa to celebrate—this was a better déjà vu! Anjali still paints and travels. Her priorities have changed, and along with her family, she is also trying to help other women who are going through what she experienced so they don't have to fight the fight alone.

2

Eat to Ease Your Symptoms

The day began great for Mrs Prasanna Menon. She was going for a mammogram and then heading out to shop with her best friend. The last few years had been hectic. Her husband, a prolific diplomat in the Indian Foreign Service (IFS), had retired. They had made Delhi their home in a predominantly IFS neighbourhood. Her regular mammogram two years ago had been normal. However, a few weeks from this check-up she had felt a lump in her breast, but because she was going through menopause at 55, she shrugged it off. Both she and her best friend got the mammogram, but she never made it to the shopping trip: her mammogram showed a cancerous growth in her breast, and just in a moment, everything changed. Memories of her childhood came rushing back. She was only 17 when her mother, a physician at PGI Chandigarh, had been diagnosed with breast cancer. She remembered the whole PGI community coming together in support of her and her sister. Her mother would eventually undergo surgery followed by radiation therapy and survive her cancer. Just as she had been supported in her childhood, in adulthood her whole neighbourhood teamed up to help her to such an extent that they even earned the nickname 'Angels of Mercy'. Advice started pouring in from all directions. However, she was very clear in her mind about her healthcare team's advice and underwent a mastectomy, which was successful with her lymph nodes being negative.

Then came the chemotherapy. The first day was uneventful; however with time the effects of the treatment began to set in. Her nails turned blue and she lost her hair, eyebrows, and eyelashes. Constipation set in and when she tried to fix it, things went overboard and she had diarrhoea. She lost the sensation for salt and things tasted bitter. Her mouth became dry and it became hard to chew on a staple like roti.

Constipation is a frequent side effect in cancer patients and is a source of great discomfort and can lead to belly pain, swelling, bloating, gas, and even nausea. In general, constipation occurs as the stool takes a longer time to travel through the large intestine (also known as the colon) which allows more water to be absorbed, leading to hard, dry stool. Interestingly, one can have constipation and diarrhoea at the same time as liquid stool can pass behind the obstructing, solid stool. Medicines like morphine (which belongs to a class of medicines called opioids) bind to receptors in the gastrointestinal system and slow down the transit time in the gut, leading to constipation. As with anything in life, it pays to be proactive as it is easier to prevent constipation than to treat it once it has occurred. Below are a few recommendations that can help with constipation:[138]

- Eating high-fibre foods, such as whole-wheat chapatti, wholegrain and bran breads/cereals, oats, fruits, vegetables, prunes, lentils, beans, peas, nuts, and seeds in meals and snacks daily can help prevent constipation.[139] There are two kinds of fibre: insoluble and soluble. Many foods contain both but are usually richer in one type than the other. Soluble fibre absorbs water, making stool softer and improving its form and consistency, which makes it easier to pass through your intestines. Examples of soluble fibre include oats, apples, beans, peas. Insoluble fibre adds bulk to your stool, easing its passage through the intestines, and can act help in the movement of material through the digestive system and helps expel stool rapidly. Examples include the skin of fruits, whole wheat flour, brown rice. Remember that the increase in fibre should be gradual and not sudden as that can result in gas, bloating, and abdominal pain.

- Drinking adequate amounts of water will also help. Patients with constipation should have a goal of eight cups of total fluids each day.[140] Try warm water and prune juice.

- Try and avoid foods and drinks that cause gas, such as cabbage and carbonated beverages.

- Avoid chewing gum and drinking with a straw as it can cause gas and abdominal discomfort.

- Above all, it is important to exercise and stay active as this can help movement of food in the gut.

Diarrhoea is, unfortunately, another side effect which is just as problematic as constipation. It can be a consequence of cancer therapy like chemotherapy, immunotherapy, radiation or even surgery if some parts of the gut are removed. Patients can also develop diarrhoea if they get infections or if the cancer itself secretes hormones. For example, a disease called the carcinoid syndrome is a serious problem as patients can become dehydrated and have electrolyte abnormalities like low potassium in the blood.

The tips below may be helpful for management of diarrhoea:[141]

- Avoid foods with high fibre, such as raw fruits and vegetables, whole grains, peas, etc which can make diarrhoea worse. Once diarrhoea subsides, you can slowly go back to foods with fibre.

- Avoid high fat and fried foods including cakes, cookies, pastries.

- Avoid alcoholic drinks, caffeine and spicy foods.

- Stay hydrated. Drink plenty (at least 8–12 cups) of non-alcoholic, non-caffeinated and non-carbonated (no fizz) beverages each day. Try drinking the majority of fluids between meals rather than with meals. Take your time, slowly sip on the fluids.

- You can lose essential electrolytes like sodium and potassium with diarrhoea. Try and eat high sodium (salted) foods like crackers and soups, broths at room temperature and high potassium foods like potatoes (without skin), bananas, papayas, and coconut water.

- Eat small, frequent meals during the day.

- It may be hard to process dairy products like milk. Try to limit your intake or avoid these foods until your diarrhoea stops. Yoghurt and buttermilk may be better tolerated.

- Try easy to digest foods like bananas, applesauce and dry toast. You can remember the acronym: The BRAT diet, which includes bananas, white rice, applesauce, and dry toast.

Dry mouth, or xerostomia, is a common complication of cancer therapy. We all have salivary glands in our mouth that secrete saliva which helps keep the mouth wet, making it easier to chew and swallow and also to prevent tooth decay. Chemotherapy, and more commonly radiation to the neck, can result in the glands not producing enough saliva, leading to xerostomia. In fact, dry mouth can persist in up to 40 per cent of patients five years after they have undergone radiation. The side effects can range from simple discomfort while chewing to infections in the gums and cavities in teeth. In addition to xerostomia, mucositis or mouth sores are a frequent complication of chemotherapy and radiation therapy, especially for patients who are undergoing therapy for head and neck cancer. It is important to be self-aware and discuss with your health care team if you are experiencing dry mouth or mouth sores and start taking these steps to keep healthy:[142]

- Good oral and dental hygiene must be followed. Gently brush your gums and teeth with a soft toothbrush after meals and before you sleep. You can rinse your mouth with a solution of baking soda (half teaspoon), salt (half teaspoon), and two cups of warm water. Use to swish and spit during the day.

- Drink plenty of fluids and always keep a water bottle handy. This will help thin the mucous and keep the body hydrated.

- Avoid dry foods and try and eat soft, moist foods that are cool or at room temperature. Moisten your food with sauces, gravy, and yoghurt. Try liquids like smoothies, lassi, and soups.

- Try sucking on sugar-free candy or sugar-free gum to help stimulate the saliva.

- Avoid acidic items including citrus fruits, foods that are dry, spicy, coarse and crunchy, and caffeinated beverages.

- Alcohol, and especially tobacco, can irritate the mouth further and should be avoided.

Mrs Menon did not let her cancer slow her down. There was minimal information on what she could eat, so she devoted her time to finding recipes in magazines, online, and any book she could lay her hands on. And alongside were the Angels of Mercy, helping out in her battle to eat nutritious food during therapy. She slowly fell into a routine: before chemotherapy she would have soup (chicken or pumpkin) and an egg sandwich. Her palate changed and she cooked a lot with coconut milk and made soft and pureed foods like stews. She experimented with food and tried to work with seasonal fruits and vegetables. Her gastronomic adventure included everything from scrambled eggs to olan (a dish from Kerela made with pumpkin, beans, and coconut milk flavoured with curry leaves). She substituted drier rotis with softer parathas. Now, more than a decade after her cancer diagnosis and treatment, she keeps herself busy with friends and family. Her foodie adventures continue and she shares recipes with other patients who are going through cancer therapy. Some of these amazing and delicious recipes can be found in this book.

THE BENEFITS OF ACUPUNCTURE

Other than diet, acupuncture has shown to be beneficial in patients with dry mouth. Deng and colleagues studied changes in the MRI of the brain in 20 healthy patients, who received real and sham acupuncture treatments. They discovered that true acupuncture led to increased production of saliva with activation of parts of the brain which was not seen in patients who received sham acupuncture treatment.[143] In a separate study, 145 cancer patients who were suffering from radiation-induced dry mouth were recruited in seven hospitals in United Kingdom.[144] One group of patients either received two oral care educational sessions for one hour, one month apart. The first section educated them on how dry mouth develops, its effects on daily living, and current research while the second session covered dietary advice and what products were available for relief from dry mouth. The second group received acupuncture sessions for 20 minutes every week for eight weeks by therapists who were all registered members of the British Acupuncture Council or equivalent bodies and attended workshops to learn the standardized protocol. Four weeks after the end of these two different types of care, the patients changed sides and received the other treatment. The results showed that the patients who received acupuncture had improvement in symptoms of dry mouth, with significant reductions in patients' reporting of severe dry mouth, sticky saliva, needing to sip liquids to swallow food, and in waking up at night to drink water. The caveat here is: refrain from trying this at home or with your neighbourhood acupuncturist. All the therapists were trained in the procedure to obtain the optimal results. Thus, it is very important to identify a reliable, trained acupuncturist.

3

The 'Chemo' Sisterhood

Before Shruti could begin her next round of chemotherapy, an unusual request came from her oncologist: would she be open to talking to someone else about her experience with chemotherapy? She wondered whom her doctor wanted her to meet. At 31, she was one of the youngest people receiving cancer chemotherapy, which she was only getting used to. The last few months had been a whirlwind. She had been holidaying in Maldives when she felt a lump in her breast on self-examination. She pushed it to the back of her mind and did not think much about it till she met a surgeon who wanted to admit her immediately for surgery the next day. Fearing the worst, she and her husband went for a second opinion when their fears were confirmed: this was cancer of the breast. Being the youngest in the family, everyone was supportive and rallied behind her, still in shock that cancer could happen to someone so young. Shruti decided early on not to let the cancer get the better of her. She refused to let it touch her spirit and refused to use a wheelchair to the operation theatre and instead walked in. Post-surgery was hard for her supportive family; her sister could not hold back her tears as she saw drains where Shruti's breast used to be.

Shruti desperately tried to get all the information she could gather regarding the side effects of chemotherapy. When she googled about it, the information was endless and overwhelming. One of the unexpected side effects of chemotherapy was the pain that she felt in her scalp when her hair started falling off. She shaved off her head and her fears of how it would change her were quickly dispelled by her husband, whose first words to her were: 'You look beautiful', and her nephew, who thought she looked 'really cool!'

With time, her hair grew back but what took time to get better was the metallic taste in her mouth, also known by its scientific name: dysgeusia. Dysgeusia is defined variably as 'an abnormal or impaired sense of taste, an unpleasant alteration of taste sensation, or a distortion or perversion of the sense of taste' and can be described as a bitter, metallic, salty, or unpleasant taste. This is closely linked to the sense of smell as both can be distorted during cancer therapy. Things can taste too salty, sugary or downright bitter. The taste changes can be measured by testing the five basic tastes: sweet, bitter, sour, salty, and umami (the savouriness of protein-rich foods) with taste strips or an instrument called ELECTROGUSTOMETER!! (That's a mouthful!!). However, the exact mechanism by which these changes occur is unknown.[145]

Possible causes include destruction of sensory receptor cells, change in the structure of the cells, and disruption of the nerve pathways in the tongue. Normal human taste bud cells turn over every 10 days and the lifespan of receptor cells in the nasal tract is about one week. These are impacted by radiation therapy and some chemotherapy agents which target and kill cells with high turnover rates. Bitter and metallic sensations can also result from the use of chemotherapeutic drugs which have compounds that are bitter and can enter the mouth through blood vessels in the posterior of the tongue—or odour receptor cells. Approximately half of patients undergoing chemotherapy only can experience dysgeusia while 66.5 per cent of patients on radiotherapy alone and 76 per cent of patients who received combined RT and CT experienced changes. While there is no specific therapy that improves outcomes, the following strategies might help improve quality of life during and after therapy:[146]

- It is important to drink plenty of liquids. Try using herbs or fruits to flavour water.

- Oral hygiene is very important. Brush your teeth and tongue after every meal and seek dental care before therapy, especially radiation for head and neck cancer.

- Freeze fresh fruits (grapes, watermelons or oranges) and snack on them.

- If you have a bad taste in the mouth, try sugar-free gum, mints or lemon drops.

- If you have a metallic taste in your mouth, avoid metallic silverware and eat in glass cups and plates and use plastic cutlery.

- Try eating foods cold or at room temperature.

- If foods taste salty or bitter, try added sweeteners like honey. If they taste too sweet, increase salty or tart flavours by adding lemon juice, vinegar, salt, and try adding citrusy foods to your overall diet.

- If food tastes bland, marinate foods to improve their flavour or add spices.

- If red meat starts tasting strange, switch to other high-protein foods such as chicken, eggs or fish.

- Strong smells can be intolerable, so try and cover beverages with a cap and sip through a straw to avoid the smell.

Shruti struggled with strong smells and food tasted too sugary. To counter this she switched to tangy foods. Golgappas and papdi chaat were her favourite comfort foods and she ate light meals and snacked a lot during chemotherapy. It was in the middle of one of these sessions when she met Neeti and a sisterhood blossomed.

Neeti is one of those people who can light up any room she walks into. She has a carefree, positive vibe about her and is always ready with a quick smile. Just like Shruti, she was only 31 when she felt a lump in her breast. Dismissing it as nothing, she slept over it and did not seek medical advice for two months. When she did go to a doctor, she had a sense of dread that this was not normal, which was confirmed when she was diagnosed with cancer. Her main memory of her surgery is how she and her husband were lay on the hospital bed watching *How I Met Your Mother*, oblivious to the world and the upcoming surgery, just holding on to each other. After the surgery came the chemotherapy, which she dreaded as her only previous exposure to it was the portrayal of cancer patients as emaciated and sick people in Bollywood movies, most of whom do not make it. (Just like Rajesh Khanna in *Anand*. If you have always wondered 'lymphosarcoma' of the intestine does not exist, it is a combination of two different cancers: lymphoma and sarcoma.) Complicating matters, she was a very sickly child and was very nauseated during pregnancy. Unfortunately, her prediction turned out to be accurate and nausea hit her hard.

Nausea and vomiting are triggered when impulses from a zone in the brain called the chemoreceptor trigger zone, and the throat and gut send a signal to the vomiting centre in the brain that something is not right. In response, the centre sends a signal to different areas in the body including the stomach, salivary centre, and nerves, resulting in vomiting. Cancer therapy causes vomiting by activating neurotransmitters. A neurotransmitter is a type of chemical messenger which transmits signals from one neuron (nerve cell) to another 'target' neuron, muscle cell, or gland cell. Subsequently, their receptors located in the chemoreceptor trigger zone, the gut and the vomiting centre are also triggered. Factors that can increase the risk for nausea and vomiting include being female, younger than 50 years of age, a history of morning sickness with past pregnancy, constipation, and if one has a tumor in the gastrointestinal tract, liver, or brain.[6] Neeti met a number of these criteria and was at high risk for chemotherapy-induced nausea and vomiting.

The nausea and vomiting can be classified into different types: acute, that happens within 24 hours after treatment starts; and delayed, which happens more than 24 hours after chemotherapy. Patients might also get anticipatory nausea and vomiting which can occur if a patient has had nausea and vomiting after an earlier chemotherapy session. This usually begins after the third or fourth treatment and is triggered by any reminder of previous times when they got sick—like the smells, sights, and sounds of the treatment room. In my practice, I have had several patients who get nauseous just from entering the chemotherapy suite or from the night before, anticipating chemotherapy the next day. Over the past decades, there has been an improvement in the control of therapy-related vomiting with the advent of several new medicines targeting active neurotransmitters in the brain and in the gut. However, there are also non-pharmacologic therapies like self-hypnosis that can potentially be of help.

Although severe vomiting needs medication, a few nutritional remedies may come in handy for patients with queasiness accompanied by little or no vomiting:[147]

- Eat five to six small meals a day and avoid keeping the stomach completely empty.[148]

- Avoid greasy and high-fat foods and consume cool, light foods which may also help reduce nauseous feelings.[149]

- Try sipping on water and other clear, cold liquids. Sip slowly. Try popsicles.

- Avoid strong food odours and try to remain outside the kitchen during food preparation if possible.[150]

- Try natural ginger tea or ginger candy. The major pharmacological activity of ginger appears to be attributed to gingerols and shogaols, biologically active secondary metabolites of ginger rhizome. Various laboratory-based and clinical studies have also shown ginger to possess anti-vomiting effects; however, the exact mechanism for anti-emetic effect is not known.

Neeti had a hard time during chemotherapy but stuck it out with the love and support of her family. She still remembers the time when she saw her three-year-old son praying for the first time: 'Meri mamma ko mere saath khila do' (God, please let my mother play with me). She tried licking a lime with salt on it to help with her nausea. Khichdi was her go-to food. The chemotherapy impacted her olfactory senses and she can no longer bear the smell of hand sanitizer. But with all struggles in life comes a silver lining: Shruti and Neeti stayed friends during and after their chemotherapy and still meet regularly. They have joined forces to help other women diagnosed with breast cancer. The Sisterhood is alive, well and thriving.

4

The 'Grape'fruit of All Evil

When you have cancer, a healthy nutritious diet is essential to keep your body strong. However, there are some food and herbal supplements that can have a detrimental effect on your health. This has gained prominence over the past decade, in part due to the explosion of oral chemotherapy. In 2005, the year I joined my fellowship in Hematology-Oncology, a majority of drugs were administered intravenously, or through IV. Patients would come to the hospital or infusion centres once or multiple times a week to get hooked onto an IV which would trickle chemotherapy in their veins over a period of minutes or hours, or even as long as for seven days continuously. Patients gave nicknames to some of these chemotherapies: for example Adriamycin, a therapy for breast cancer, was frequently referred to as the 'Red Devil' for its deep red colour and for the side effects it caused: nausea, vomiting, hair loss, and heart failure, amongst other things.

This trend has changed rapidly with oral chemotherapies being used to treat all kinds of diseases from lung, liver, and breast cancers to even certain blood cancers. Patients can dose themselves at home and follow up at intervals with their oncologist with lab work to make sure their body is tolerating the side effects of this therapy. Along with the convenience of oral chemotherapies comes the possibility of interactions with food. This is because the 'drug' undergoes several modifications by the body, the first of which are liberation (release of the drug from its formulation: for example, a capsule), and absorption (from the stomach or other parts of the gastrointestinal tract into the circulation). This can be impacted by food and other factors like fat content in the meal. For example, the absorption of Nilotinib (therapy for Chronic Myeloid Leukemia) and Lapatinib (for patients with breast cancer) is increased when administered with food and so it is recommended to administer these on an empty stomach. There are also a group of enzymes called the Cytochrome P (CYP) that play a critical role in how drugs are broken down in the body. The levels of these enzymes can be impacted by herbal supplements and various foods including the relatively sour grapefruit and seville (sour) oranges which can inhibit activity of CYP3A4, thus increasing the levels of the chemotherapy in the body. This can lead to unintended side effects and increased toxicity from the drug administered. On the other hand, some herbal agents can increase the breakdown of chemotherapy, leading it to be potentially less effective.

Moral of the story: In addition to focusing on what to eat during therapy, it is also critical to know what to avoid. In the end it comes down to communication with your healthcare team so they are aware of your dietary habits and supplements use and can guide you on when is the best time in the day to take oral chemotherapy.

INTERMITTENT FASTING: FAD OR FOREVER

Fasting has long been a part of India culture, with calorie restriction for a period of days or some chosen days of the week being widely prevalent.

Recently, though, the concept of 'intermittent fasting' has gained traction where the focus is on the time frame within which food is eaten. This concept can be traced back to prehistoric times, when farming was non-existent and humans survived long periods before eating, as it took a lot of time to hunt and gather food. This was also the case in the not-so-distant past, with people going to bed early as there were very few distractions to stay awake. However, with the advent of 24/7 entertainment, this has changed dramatically. We now snack till the wee hours of the morning, binging on our favourite show(s) *(guilty as charged: why did they have to make* Game of Thrones *so engrossing???).*

There are different variations in intermittent fasting; time restricted fasting (for example the 16:8 method in which you consume your calories in eight hour and fast for the other 16), alternate day fasting and 5:2 where you eat normal over five days and limit yourself to one 500-600 calorie meal on the other two days. Intermittent fasting has been postulated to be beneficial for multiple health conditions like obesity, insulin resistance and cardiovascular diseases.[151] In cancer, the potential benefit has largely been confined to mouse models in the laboratory that have demonstrated benefit in combination of fasting with chemotherapy, but not as a stand-alone intervention. Clinical trials in humans have focused on compliance with fasting, predominantly in patients with breast and prostate cancer. For example, forty overweight or obese, newly diagnosed prostate cancer patients who elected prostate surgery were randomized to a trial of daily caloric restriction.[152] This demonstrated an adherence rate in 95 per cent of patients who did not have any significant adverse events. However, the results were mixed in a trial which was more rigorous with calorie control. In a Dutch trial, women with breast cancer were randomized to receive either a fasting mimicking diet (FMD) or their regular diet for three days prior to and during neoadjuvant chemotherapy (chemotherapy administered before potential surgery).[153] Patients received six or eight cycles of neoadjuvant chemotherapy. The FMD was a four-day plant-based low amino-acid substitution diet, consisting of soups, broths, liquids and tea with the goal of calorie content decrease from day 1 (~1200 kcal), to days 2–4 (~200 kcal). Though the investigators did not find a difference in toxicity between both groups, the rate of adherence to FMD was low with 81.5 per cent patients completing the first cycle, approximately 50 per cent completing two cycles, 33.8 per cent at least four cycles and only 20.0 per cent of the patients complied during all cycles of chemotherapy. This points to the challenge of intermittent fasting during cancer therapy which should only be attempted in the context of a clinical trial with a care team of physicians and nutritionists. The application of intermittent fasting in cancer patients can also be a cause of concern as it could result in cachexia, anorexia and lead to malnutrition in patients who are already frail and nutritionally compromised.

No studies have determined whether intermittent fasting has any effect on cancer recurrence or on cancer prevention, though short-term FMD was shown to reduce abdominal obesity and markers of inflammation, indicating that periodic use of an FMD could potentially have preventive effects for obesity-related cancers[154].

So, the right question may not be 'to eat or not to eat', but rather 'when to eat'. And remember, this does not give you a carte blanche to binge on unhealthy food during the non-fasting period. Stick to eating healthy by cooking up some of the recipes listed by our amazingly talented contributors.

Recipes

CONTRIBUTED BY PRASANNA MENON, PUSHPESH PANT AND
ANITA JAISINGHANIA

Sago (Sabudana) Khichdi

Serves 4

Preparation time: Overnight soaking; 5 minutes for chopping and grinding

Cooking time: 15 minutes

INGREDIENTS

250 gm sabudana
1 onion, finely chopped
1 potato, boiled and cut into small pieces
2 tbsp oil
1 tsp cumin seeds
1 cup peanuts, crushed
1 green chilli, finely chopped
1 large bunch of coriander leaves, finely chopped
Salt to taste

INSTRUCTIONS

Wash and soak the sabudana for 3–4 hours. Water should cover the sabudana for soaking. Drain and leave overnight to drain completely. In a kadhai, heat the oil and sauté the cumin and onion till soft. Add the potato and stir. Mix the salt and crushed peanuts into the sabudana. Add this into the kadhai and stir gently till it is well mixed into the onion and potato. Add the green chilli and coriander and stir again to mix. Cover and cook for 3–5 minutes on a low flame till the sabudana turns translucent. Take the pan off the heat and allow it to rest for a few minutes. Serve hot.

NOTES

While stirring and mixing, take care that the sabudana does not get mashed.

Tomato Chutney

Serves 8–10
Preparation time: 5 minutes
Cooking time: 15-20 minutes

INGREDIENTS

8 medium-sized tomatoes, finely chopped
2 tbsp sesame oil (coconut oil, olive oil or good quality vegetable oil can also be used)
1 tsp mustard seeds
2 garlic cloves, finely chopped
2–3 tbsp sugar or gur (jaggery) to taste
A sprig of curry leaves
1 tsp red chilli powder
1 tsp black pepper powder
1 tsp cinnamon powder
Salt to taste

INSTRUCTIONS

Heat the oil in a kadhai or saucepan. Add mustard seeds and heat till the seeds splutter. Add the curry leaves and garlic and fry for a minute or till the garlic turns golden. Add the tomatoes, salt, and remaining spices. Cover and cook on a low heat till most of the liquid runs dry. Now, add the sugar or gur and simmer for a few minutes more till the chutney is almost dry, making sure the sugar does not burn. Remove from heat and serve. This chutney will stay refrigerated for a week or so and is good in sandwiches with cheese.

Green Papaya Salad

Serves 6–8

Preparation time: 10 minutes

INGREDIENTS

1 green papaya, peeled and grated

2 cucumbers, peeled and cut into small cubes

2 medium onions, sliced

1–2 green chillies, finely chopped

½ cup vinegar

2 tbsp sugar

1 tsp salt

1 large bunch of coriander leaves, finely chopped

1 cup peanuts, crushed

INSTRUCTIONS

Stir the sugar, salt, and green chillies into the vinegar till the sugar dissolves. Mix the papaya, cucumber, and onion well and add the vinegar mixture. Mix well and add the chopped coriander. Chill well. Before serving, mix in the crushed peanuts.

Sweet and Sour Pumpkin Bharta

Serves 4–6

Preparation time: 10 minutes

Cooking time: 15–20 minutes

INGREDIENTS

200 gm yellow pumpkin, peeled and chopped into medium-sized pieces

1 tsp cumin seeds

2–3 tbsp oil (use sesame or coconut oil for extra flavour)

1 onion, finely chopped

1 green chilli, finely chopped

1 tsp red chilli flakes (optional)

1 tsp turmeric powder

1 tbsp vinegar

1 tbsp sugar

½ cup water

A sprig of curry leaves

A few coriander leaves, chopped

Salt to taste

INSTRUCTIONS

In a kadhai or saucepan heat the oil. Add the cumin and onion pieces and sauté till the onion is soft. Now add the chopped pumpkin, salt, chilli, turmeric, and water and cook covered on a low heat till the pumpkin is soft. Mash the pumkin mixture roughly and add the sugar, vinegar, and coriander and curry leaves. Cover and cook for 5 minutes or so on a low heat.

Serve with roti or rice.

NOTES

For added creaminess, mix in a little coconut milk powder and heat for a minute or so.

Olan

Serves 6-8

Preparation time: Overnight soaking; 5 minutes for peeling and chopping

Cooking time: 20-25 minutes

INGREDIENTS

200–250 gm yellow pumpkin, peeled and chopped into large pieces (2–3 inches)

½ cup black eyed beans

1 packet coconut milk powder or 1 can coconut milk

1 green chilli, slit and sliced lengthwise

½ inch ginger, chopped

1 cup water

A handful of curry leaves

Salt to taste

INSTRUCTIONS

Soak beans overnight. Drain and rinse. Put the pumpkin pieces, beans, salt, ginger, green chilli, curry leaves, and water into a pressure cooker and cook till done (approximately 10 minutes after cooker comes to full pressure). Once the cooker cools, open it and add the coconut milk. Simmer on low heat for a minute or so. Check seasoning and take off from the heat. Serve with rice or bread.

NOTES

This is like a stew. For more flavour, stir in a spoon of coconut oil before serving.

Lauki Morkootu
(Bottlegourd in Yoghurt)

Serves 4

Preparation time: 5 minutes

Cooking time: 10–15 minutes

INGREDIENTS

250 gm lauki

1 tsp turmeric

1 tsp mustard seeds

1 tbsp oil

1 green chilli, sliced into two

A handful of curry leaves

1 cup yoghurt

½ cup water

Salt to taste

INSTRUCTIONS

Peel and chop the lauki into medium-sized pieces. In a kadhai or saucepan, heat the oil and fry the mustard seeds till they pop. Add the curry leaves, lauki, green chilli, salt, haldi and water. Cover and cook on low heat till the lauki pieces are soft and well-cooked. Beat the yoghurt and add to the cooked vegetable mixture. Stir well and remove from heat before the yoghurt separates. Cool and serve with rice.

Chicken Stew

Serves 4

Preparation time: 10 minutes

Cooking time: 20–30 minutes

INGREDIENTS

200–250 gm chicken thighs

1 medium potato, peeled and quartered

1 onion, sliced

1 capsicum, cut into 8 pieces

2 tbsp coconut oil

1 inch piece cinnamon

1 small piece star anise

3–4 cloves

3–4 peppercorns

1 tsp fennel seeds

1 bay leaf

A handful of curry leaves

2 green chillies, sliced into two

1 packet coconut milk powder or 1 can coconut milk

1 cup water

Salt to taste

INSTRUCTIONS

Skin and chop the chicken thighs into three pieces. Heat the oil in a kadhai or saucepan, add the spices and fry for a minute or so. Add the curry leaves, chicken pieces, vegetables, and green chilli. Sauté for 3–4 minutes. Add salt and water, cover and cook on low heat till the chicken is well-cooked. Add the coconut milk and bring to a simmer for a few minutes. Take off from the heat and serve with rice, paratha or bread.

Chicken Stir-Fry

Serves 4-6
Preparation time: 10 minutes
Cooking time: 15 minutes

INGREDIENTS

250 gm boneless chicken, cut into bite-sized pieces
1 large onion, sliced into 8 pieces
1 capsicum, sliced into strips
½ cup cashew or walnuts, roasted
1 tbsp soya sauce
1 tbsp vinegar
1 tbsp honey
1 green chilli, sliced
1 tsp black pepper powder
3 tbsp sesame oil
A handful coriander leaves and basil, chopped
Salt to taste

INSTRUCTIONS

Heat the oil. Add chicken pieces, onion, and capsicum and sauté for a few minutes. Cover and cook, stirring from time to time till the chicken is done. Add the soya sauce, vinegar, honey, herbs, and salt and stir well. Add the nuts and heat for a minute. Serve hot with noodles or rice.

Chana with Lime and Garlic

Serves 4–6

Preparation time: 5 minutes

Cooking time: 20–30 minutes (time to cook the chana)

INGREDIENTS

1 cup white chana (chickpea)

2 garlic cloves, finely chopped

2 tbsp grated fresh coconut (optional)

1 tsp salt

1 cup water

2 tbsp sesame oil

1 tsp mustard seeds

A handful of curry leaves

1 dried red chilli (optional)

1 green chilli, sliced

A handful of basil, mint, and coriander leaves, chopped

Juice of 1 lemon

½ tsp sugar

INSTRUCTIONS

Soak the chana overnight. Drain and rinse. Boil the chana with salt and water in a pressure cooker till soft. Drain and keep aside. In a kadhai or saucepan heat the oil and add the mustard seeds. When they pop add the red chilli, curry leaves, and garlic and fry for a few minutes till the garlic is golden. Add the chana, green chilli, sugar, and green herbs and sauté well for a few minutes. Take off the heat and mix in the fresh coconut and lime juice. Serve as a warm salad.

Rice Undas
(Steamed Rice Balls)

Makes 20–25 dumplings
Preparation time: 5 minutes
Cooking time: 20–25 minutes

INGREDIENTS

1 cup rice powder
2 cups water
2 tbsp coconut oil
1 tsp salt
1 tsp sugar
1 tsp red chilli flakes
1 green chilli, finely chopped
A handful of curry leaves and coriander leaves, finely chopped
1 onion, finely chopped

INSTRUCTIONS

Heat the oil in a kadhai or saucepan and sauté the onion till golden. Add chilli flakes, salt, sugar, green chilli, green herbs, and water and bring to a boil. Add the rice powder stirring all the time and cook, stirring well till the water is absorbed and a dough is formed which leaves the side of the pan. Cool slightly. While still hot, form into balls and steam in a steamer for 10 minutes. Remove and serve with tomato or coconut chutney. These rice balls can be used as dumplings in a stew or soup.

Semiya Idli

Makes 16 idlis
Preparation time: Overnight for soaking
Cooking time: 15–20 minutes

INGREDIENTS

1 cup sooji (semolina)
1 cup unroasted semiya (thicker variety)
2 tbsp ghee or butter
½ cup yoghurt
½ cup milk
1 cup water, water for the batter
½ cup cashew, crushed
1 tbsp oil
1 tsp mustard seeds
1 green chilli, chopped
A handful of curry leaves, chopped
1 tbsp ginger, grated
1 tbsp Eno Salt or baking powder
Salt to taste

INSTRUCTIONS

Lightly roast the sooji and keep aside. Fry the semiya in the butter or ghee till golden. Mix the semiya and sooji and add the yoghurt, milk, water, and salt. Stir well and leave overnight. Heat the oil and fry the mustard seeds till they pop. Add the cashew nuts and fry till golden. Add this to the semiya mixture along with the green chilli, ginger, and curry leaves. Add water until the consistency is similar to idli batter. Mix in the Eno or baking powder, stir well, and steam in a greased idli mould for 10 minutes. Cool and remove from the mould. Serve with coconut chutney.

Kanda Poha

Serves 6

Preparation time: 35 minutes

Cooking time: 15 minutes

INGREDIENTS

2 cups poha, thicker variety

2 tbsp oil

1 onion, finely chopped

1 tsp cumin seeds

½ cup green peas

1 medium-sized potato, boiled and cut into small pieces

1 tsp sugar

1 tsp turmeric powder

1 green chilli, chopped finely

A handful of coriander leaves, chopped

Juice of one lemon

Bhujia or sev (Haldiram's bhujia is good)

Salt to taste

INSTRUCTIONS

Wash the poha gently, drain and let it rest for around 30 minutes. In a kadhai or saucepan heat the oil. Add the cumin and onion and sauté till the onion is soft. Add the peas and potato and cook covered on low heat till the peas are done (about five minutes or so). Mix the drained poha well with the haldi, salt, sugar, green chilli, and coriander. Add this mixture to the kadhai. Stir well, cover, and cook on low heat for 5 minutes or so till the poha is soft and done. Cool and squeeze the lemon juice over the poha. Sprinkle bhujia and serve.

Papaya/Mango and Honey Smoothie

Serves 2

Preparation time: 15 minutes

INGREDIENTS

1 cup papaya/mango, diced

1 cup hung yoghurt

1 tbsp oats

1 tbsp honey

½ tbsp pistachio flakes, for garnish

A pinch of saffron threads (soaked in lukewarm milk), for garnish

INSTRUCTIONS

Put all ingredients in a blender and mix till a thick consistency is obtained. Pour the smoothie into glasses and garnish with pistachio slivers and strands of saffron.

Date/Fig Smoothie

Serves 2

Preparation time: 15 minutes

INGREDIENTS

1 cup dates, deseeded (or dried figs soaked in milk overnight)

1 banana, ripe but not soft

2 cups hung yoghurt

1 tbsp fresh cream (optional)

½ tbsp crushed almonds, pistachio flakes and edible flowers, for garnish

INSTRUCTIONS

Put the chopped bananas and dates/figs in a mixer, add yoghurt and cream and blend into a smooth paste. Pour into glasses. Garnish with pistachio flakes, almonds, and edible flowers.

Unripe and Ripe Mango Smoothie

Serves 2
Preparation time: 30 minutes

INGREDIENTS

1 cup ripe mango, cubed
½ cup raw mango, cubed
1 tsp honey (optional)
1 tsp fennel seeds
½ tsp black pepper powder
10 mint leaves
2 cups fresh yoghurt
A pinch of black rock salt (kala namak)
Aam papad, thinly sliced, for garnish

INSTRUCTIONS

In a saucepan, add mangoes and fennel seeds. Cook for 2 minutes. Keep aside and allow the mix to cool down completely. Stir in the honey. Add in a mixer along with the remaining ingredients. Blend for 20 seconds. Pour into glasses and garnish with thin slices of aam papad.

Sweet Corn Smoothie

Serves 2

Preparation time: 15 minutes

INGREDIENTS

1 cup creamy sweet corn

2 cups fresh yoghurt

1 tsp dried pomegranate seeds, powdered

½ tsp cumin seeds, powdered

A pinch of black rock salt

Fresh pomegranate seeds (for garnishing)

Prunes/dried or stewed apricots (for garnishing)

INSTRUCTIONS

Put all ingredients in a mixer and blend. Garnish with fresh pomegranate seeds and prunes/dried or stewed apricots.

Ginger Smoothie

Serves 2

Preparation time: 7–8 minutes

INGREDIENTS

1 cup hung yoghurt

A pinch of black rock salt

A pinch of cumin seeds, roasted

A pinch of fennel seed powder

2 tsp ginger, chopped

½ tsp dried ginger powder

1 tsp sugar, powdered

½ tsp black peppercorns (optional)

1 tbsp fresh cream

A small sprig of mint leaves

INSTRUCTIONS

Put all the ingredients in a blender except the cream. Add ¼ cup of water and mix well. Pour in glasses and top with a little cream. Sprinkle a pinch of powdered fennel seeds and dried ginger powder. Serve after garnishing with fresh mint leaves.

Green Gram (Whole Moong) Soup

Serves 3–4

Preparation time: 10 minutes

Cooking time: 20 minutes

INGREDIENTS

1 cup whole moong dal, unhusked, picked, and washed

1 medium onion, peeled and finely chopped

1 two-inch piece of ginger, chopped

1 green chilli, chopped

1 tomato, finely chopped

½ tsp cumin seeds, coarsely ground

A small sprig of coriander leaves, chopped

½ tbsp black peppercorn, coarsely ground

Salt to taste

INSTRUCTIONS

Drain the moong and put into a medium pan with about 4 cups of water. Add the onion, ginger, green chilli, tomato, and crushed cumin seeds. Cook for about 20 minutes or till the green gram is well done. Mash the green gram well with the ladle and add some more water till it becomes soupy. Add the salt and mix well. Serve hot, garnished with coriander leaves and crushed black pepper.

Yellow Pumpkin Soup

Serves 4
Preparation time: 10 minutes
Cooking time: 20 minutes

INGREDIENTS

2½ cups yellow pumpkin, washed, chopped with skin into discs
1 large onion, roughly chopped
2 green chillies
1 inch piece of ginger
2 garlic cloves
¼ tsp roasted cumin seeds
10 curry leaves, finely chopped (for garnishing)
Salt to taste

INSTRUCTIONS

Put the yellow pumpkin in a pressure cooker along with the onion, green chillies, ginger, garlic, roasted cumin seeds, and 2 cups water. Pressure cook for about 10 minutes. Take off the weight and cool. Put into a blender. After it is well blended put it back on heat and bring to boil. Season to taste. Serve hot, garnished with curry leaves.

Mulligatawny Soup

Serves 2–3

Cooking time: 30 minutes

INGREDIENTS

1 tsp coriander seeds

1 tsp cumin seeds

½ tsp black peppercorns

1 dry red chilli

3–4 garlic cloves, crushed

1 tsp ginger, scraped and sliced

1½ tsp butter

½ tsp fenugreek seeds

6–8 curry leaves

1 tomato, sliced

2 tsp lime juice

Oil for cooking

Salt to taste

INSTRUCTIONS

Grind the coriander seeds, cumin seeds, black peppercorns, dry red chilli, garlic, and ginger into a coarse paste. Keep aside. Heat the oil in a pot. Add the fenugreek seeds and sauté till brown. Add the curry leaves and then add the ground paste. Fry till slightly brown. Add the tomato and about 4 cups water. Cook until the mixture thickens. Add the lime juice. Season to taste and serve hot.

Green Gram (Whole Moong) Pancake

Serves 4

Preparation time: Overnight soaking; 45 minutes

Cooking time: 10-15 minutes

INGREDIENTS

For the batter:
1 cup whole moong dal
2 tbsp Bengal gram (chickpeas)
1 tbsp rice flour
Salt to taste

For the topping:
½ onion, finely chopped
1 inch piece of ginger, finely chopped
1 green chilli, deseeded and finely chopped
1tbsp grated coconut
A sprig of fresh coriander/mint leaves

INSTRUCTIONS

Soak the moong and gram lentils overnight. Drain and blend to obtain a smooth batter of dropping consistency. Add a little water if required. Transfer to a large bowl. Add rice flour to get extra crispiness in your dosas. Also, add salt to taste. Pour a ladleful of the batter on a hot griddle. Spread it in a circular motion. Sprinkle a few drops of ghee or oil along with finely chopped onion, cumin, ginger, and chilli over the pancake. Flip to cook both sides evenly. Serve with thick, naturally sweet yoghurt or coconut milk.

Pressed Rice with Vegetables, Eggs and Cottage Cheese

Serves 2

Preparation time: 15 minutes

Cooking time: 20 minutes

INGREDIENTS

50 gm pressed rice flakes (poha), drenched in water in a colander, then spread out gently to dry

1 tsp vegetable oil

½ tsp mustard seeds

¼ tsp turmeric powder

½ tsp Kashmiri red chilli powder

½ tsp garam masala, optional

50 gm cauliflower, broken into florets

1 boiled potato/egg cut into wedges

50 gm French beans, stringed and cut

2 medium carrots, scraped and grated

50 gm green peas, shelled and lightly boiled

2 medium tomatoes, quartered

50 gm cottage cheese, cubed

1 tbsp sugar

1 tbsp lemon juice

2–3 green chillies, deseeded

A large sprig of coriander leaves (for garnishing)

1 inch piece of ginger, scraped and cut in thin strips (for garnishing)

Salt to taste

INSTRUCTIONS

Heat the oil in a large, flat pan. Add the mustard seeds and the powdered spices. Mix well for 30 seconds. Add the pressed rice, mixing lightly with a flat spatula. Reduce heat to very low and remove from heat after about a minute. In another pan, heat some more butter and brown the cauliflower. Then stir-fry the potatoes, French beans, carrots, and peas. Add the tomatoes and cook till the tomatoes are just scalded. Add the cottage cheese in the end, if using. Stir in the sugar, salt, and lemon juice along with the green chillies. Arrange in layers in a serving dish, alternating the pressed rice flakes and vegetables and placing the potato or egg wedges on the periphery. Serve hot, garnished with coriander leaves and ginger.

Honey-Laced 'Pongal'

Serves 2
Preparation time: 15 minutes
Cooking time: 25 minutes

INGREDIENTS

½ cup whole moong dal
½ cup small grain rice
½ cup milk
1 tbsp oats
1 tbsp honey (or more to taste)
1 tbsp ghee/butter
¼ cup raisins
6–8 black peppercorns
1 clove
2–3 green cardamoms
1 tsp almond flakes

INSTRUCTIONS

Dry roast moong dal till it releases an aroma. Roast oats and rice separately. Heat ghee/butter in a pan. Add peppercorns, clove, cardamoms, and raisins. Stir-fry briskly for 20 seconds. Put in rice, oats, and moong dal along with 3 cups of water and ½ cup of milk. Boil or pressure cook till the mixture reaches porridge consistency. Stir in honey after the mixture cools. Garnish with almond flakes.

Floral Fudge
(Parijat Kalakand)

Serves 4

Preparation time: 20 minutes (including time taken for boiling milk to reduce and thicken)

Cooking time: 20 minutes

INGREDIENTS

1 cup jasmine flowers, washed well and soaked in 1 cup of milk overnight

200 gm paneer, crumbled

100 gm milk powder

Sugar, powdered, to taste

¼ tsp green cardamom powder

1 tsp pistachio slivers

INSTRUCTIONS

Drain flowers from the milk. Reserve. In a bowl, mix well the paneer, milk powder, and sugar. Slowly add the milk in which the flowers were soaked. Take care to add just enough milk to keep the mixture moist. Sprinkle some flowers on top and place in the fridge to set. Sprinkle cardamom powder and pistachio slivers on top before serving.

Daily Morning Chai

Serves 2

Preparation time: 5 minutes

INGREDIENTS

2 black tea bags (preferably PG Tips, an English brand)

12 almonds

4 slices fresh ginger

2 tsp honey

2 tbsp warm milk or your preferred nut milk

INSTRUCTIONS

In two mugs, put a tea bag, 6 almonds, 2 slices of ginger, and 1 tsp of honey each. Pour water over each cup, leaving some space at the top for milk. Let it steep for 3 minutes. Squeeze out the tea leaves and pour 1 tbsp of milk into each cup. At this point, you may leave the ginger in or take it out. Leaving it in will continue to increase the flavour. After you have finished your tea, peel the almonds, discard the peel, and eat the almonds.

NOTES

This is a simple home chai. No brewing or cooking is required. It can be had straight out of a kettle.

Cheese Toast

Serves 4

Preparation time: 20 minutes

INGREDIENTS

8 slices sandwich bread

2 tomatoes, minced

½ cup onion, minced

2 tbsp fresh coriander, chopped

1 green chili, minced

1 tsp toasted ground cumin seeds

1½ cups grated melting cheese

Ghee, to cook

INSTRUCTIONS

Lay 4 slices of bread flat on a surface. Spread the tomatoes, onion, coriander, green chili, cumin seeds, and cheese on top evenly. Top each with another piece of bread and cook the sandwiches on both sides in a warm skillet using ghee until the cheese has melted and the sandwich is golden brown on both sides. Serve immediately. This toast is best served with sweet mango chutney. This cheese toast can be made with Amul cheese and is delicious with a cup of masala chai.

NOTES

Cook the sandwiches open faced in an oven. Add crumbled bacon to the sandwiches.

Chicken Pakoras with Mint Chutney

Serves 4

Cooking time: 30 minutes plus time for marinating

INGREDIENTS

For the pakoras:

2 chicken breasts, boneless and skinless

2 tbsp plain yogurt

1 tsp minced garlic

½ tsp chili powder

½ tsp turmeric

2 tsp salt, divided

For the batter:

1 cup besan (chickpea flour)

1 tsp ajwain

1 tsp black pepper powder

For frying:

2–3 cups frying oil (canola, sunflower or peanut)

1 egg, lightly whisked

For the mint chutney:

1 apple, cored and diced

1 green chilli pepper, whole (optional)

½ cup yoghurt

¼ cup roasted peanuts

1 tsp salt

Juice from 1 lemon

1 cup mint leaves, loosely packed

1 bunch fresh coriander, bottom 3 inches removed

INSTRUCTIONS

To make the pakoras:
Trim the fat from the chicken breasts and marinate them in yoghurt, garlic, chilli powder, turmeric, and 1 tsp salt. Set aside in the refrigerator for 2–4 hours or overnight. Toss the chickpea flour with ajwain, 1 tsp salt, and black pepper in a shallow container. Slice the chicken breasts each into 6–8 long slices. Pour the egg over the chicken strips to evenly coat. Dredge each chicken piece in the chickpea mixture until coated evenly. Heat the oil in a shallow frying pan. When it is hot, gently add the chicken pieces. Cook on each side for 2-3 minutes or until lightly brown and firm. Serve immediately with mint chutney.

To make the mint chutney:
In a blender, combine apple, green chilli, yoghurt, peanuts, salt, and lemon juice and blend until smooth. Add the mint leaves in two to three parts, followed by the fresh coriander and blend until smooth. Refrigerate until ready to serve.

Chickpea Chilla with Avocado Masala

Serves 2–4
Cooking time: 30 minutes

INGREDIENTS

For the chickpea chilla:
¼ cup chickpea flour (besan)
4 tbsp olive oil
2 extra large eggs
2–3 tbsp yoghurt
A pinch of turmeric
A pinch of black pepper powder

A pinch of salt
1 tbsp olive oil
Red radish, sliced (for garnishing)

For the avocado masala:
1 large avocado or 2 small
2 tbsp chopped fresh coriander leaves
½ small green chilli, minced
1 tsp coriander seeds
Juice from ½ lemon
A pinch of salt
2 tsp sesame seeds

INSTRUCTIONS

To make the avocado masala:
Mash the avocado and add the coriander leaves, minced green chilli, coriander seeds, lemon and salt. Whip together until desired texture is achieved.

To make the chickpea chilla:
Whisk the chickpea flour, olive oil, eggs, yoghurt, turmeric, black pepper, and salt together until smooth. Heat up a non-stick pan with 1 tbsp of olive oil and swirl the oil around to coat the pan. Drop in small mounds of the chilla batter. Within 2 minutes, gently test the edges of the chillas with a spatula and when the bottom appears to be done, flip them over and cook for another minute or two. Spread avocado masala on top, sprinkle with sesame seeds, garnish with sliced radish, and serve.

NOTES

The chilla is a savoury pancake made with chickpea flour. It takes minutes to make, is deeply flavourful and can be made in many different ways. You can also top this up with peanut butter, Indian pickles and yoghurt. The crowning glory here, avocado masala, is nutritious and tasty. Using a rolling pin, lightly crush the coriander seeds for the avocado masala; they will release more lemon flavour. Chickpea may be replaced with millet or amaranth flour to make the pancake vegan. Leave the egg out and add 2 tablespoons of almond or other nut milk.

Sapodilla Rice Pudding
(Chikoo Kheer)

Serves 3

Preparation time : 1 hour or more for soaking

INGREDIENTS

½ cup basmati rice

3 cups milk

½ cup sugar

¼ tsp cardamom, ground

2 cups chikoo, pureed

INSTRUCTIONS

Rinse the basmati rice 3 times. Then, cover in cool water and soak for 30 minutes. Drain and set aside. In a stockpot on low-medium heat, begin to reduce the milk. Stir frequently to prevent a layer from forming on top. Once it is reduced by half, add the drained rice and sugar. Cook covered for 8–10 minutes until most of the liquid is absorbed by the rice. When the rice is 1–2 minutes from being done, add the cardamom and stir. Let the kheer sit covered for 10–15 minutes. Gently fold the chikoo puree in the kheer. Serve warm.

NOTES

Serve with chopped pistachios on top. You can make kheer with your favourite fruit puree, such as mango or strawberry puree, instead of chikoo. Make this vegan by replacing regular milk with coconut or almond milk. Consistency may vary.

Cucumber Raita

Serves 3
Preparation time: 15 minutes

INGREDIENTS

2 medium cucumbers (or 1 large cucumber), minced
½ small red onion, minced
1 apple, minced
2 cups plain yoghurt
1 tsp cumin, ground
1 tsp salt
3 tsp olive oil
1 tsp mustard seeds

INSTRUCTIONS

Mix the cucumbers, onion, and apple. Whisk the yoghurt in a large bowl with the salt and cumin. Then, fold in the chopped cucumbers, onion, and apple. Heat up the oil and pop the mustard seeds. Fold into the raita and refrigerate until ready to serve. The raita can be kept in the refrigerator for 2–3 days. It will keep for 2–3 days in the refrigerator. Onion and cucumbers generate a lot of water. If you notice the raita getting watery, simply drain. Add lemon juice or lemon zest for added brightness.

NOTES

This recipe shows you just how simple a raita can be. Red onion and a vegetable is all it takes. Feel free to make some additions with whatever you have in your fridge. Substitute red onion with green onion.

Fruit Custard

Serves 4–6

Preparation time: 20 minutes

One of the best ways to utilize the bounty of summer fruit, especially berries, mangoes, and peaches, is by making a fragrant home-made custard. A hit with children and adults alike, it can be infused with vanilla, cardamom, cinnamon, nutmeg or rose water.

INGREDIENTS

2 cups whole milk

2 cups heavy cream

Ginger, unpeeled and chopped into 2-inch pieces

1 large whole cinnamon stick

1 tbsp green cardamom pods, crushed

A pinch of saffron threads

A pinch of salt

3 tbsp cornstarch

¾ cup sugar

2 whole large eggs

50 gm butter

INSTRUCTIONS

In a stockpot, combine the milk, cream, ginger, cinnamon, and cardamom pods and bring the mixture to a boil. Simmer for

7–10 minutes. Then, turn the heat off and let the mixture rest for 5 minutes. Strain and stir in the saffron threads and salt. Whisk together the sugar and the cornstarch in a bowl. Add the eggs and whisk together. Add some of the hot milk into the bowl and mix until smooth. Pour it back in with the rest of the milk and continue whisking over medium heat until the custard is thick and light. Be careful not to over-boil—bubbles should not get vigorous. Take it off the heat and let it cool for 10 minutes. Stir it occasionally to prevent film from forming on top. Cut the butter into tablespoon-size portions and whisk it into the cream. Always make sure it is smoothly incorporated before you add the next tablespoon of butter. Cover with plastic wrap and refrigerate until further use.

NOTES

To make the custard lighter, eliminate the heavy cream and use 4 cups of milk instead. Replace the cardamom and cinnamon with vanilla or other spices. Custard will keep well in the refrigerator for up to 5 days; however, add fruit no more than 2–3 hours before serving it. Add sliced almonds or other nuts as a crunchy topping.

Fruit Chaat

Serves 4
Preparation time: 15 minutes

INGREDIENTS

½ cucumber
½ pineapple
¼ seedless watermelon
1 mango
2 tbsp mint leaves, finely chopped

1 tsp chaat masala, or a pinch of cumin, ground, a pinch of black salt, and a pinch of chilli powder

INSTRUCTIONS

Cut the cucumber lengthwise into quarters, then chop into half-inch pieces. Remove the rind from the pineapple and then chop into half-inch pieces. Cut the watermelon into half-inch cubes. Peel the mango and dice into quarter-inch pieces. Combine the fruits together, gently stir to evenly distribute. Sprinkle the top with mint leaves and chaat masala (or cumin, black salt, and chilli powder). Chill and serve. The combination of sweet, spicy, salty, and fresh makes this a perfect summer snack.

NOTES

Add sesame seeds or sunflower seeds for texture.

Honey–Lime Soda

Serves 2
Preparation time: 5 minutes

INGREDIENTS

2 limes
2 tbsp honey
2 tbsp warm water
2 cups soda water
A pinch of salt
Ice

INSTRUCTIONS

This is a take on the classic fresh lime soda we've all enjoyed growing up. Squeeze the juice from the two limes into two glasses. Drizzle one tablespoon of honey into each glass and pour some warm water over it to just dissolve the honey. Pour soda water, stir, add ice, and serve.

Khichdi

Serves 6
Preparation and Cooking time: 2 hours + time for soaking

INGREDIENTS

½ cup (100 gm) channa dal
1 cup (200 gm) basmati rice
1 tsp turmeric
1 tsp black pepper
½ tsp ground cloves
1 tsp salt
3 tbsp ghee or oil
Poached or fried egg, nuts, dry fruits or fresh herbs (optional, as toppings)

INSTRUCTIONS

Rinse the rice and lentil mix in water twice. Soak for 3 minutes. Drain by pouring most of the water out. A little water remaining is okay. Combine the mix with the turmeric, black pepper, ground cloves, and salt. Add 5 cups of water and bring to a boil. Lower the heat, cover the stockpot, and simmer for 1½ hours on low heat, stirring every 15–20 minutes to make sure it is not sticking to the bottom. The mixture should be thick and creamy. Drizzle ghee on top and serve.

NOTES

Every region, and possibly home, boasts its own version of khichdi using different combinations of grains and beans. It may be eaten for breakfast, lunch or dinner!

Add 2 cups of finely chopped or grated carrots or squash to the mixture in the last 10 minutes of cooking.

Add 4 cups of chopped fresh spinach at the end of cooking (just before turning the heat off and adding the ghee). It will wilt but retain its colour.

Saffron Morning Halwa

Serves 4
Cooking time: 15 minutes

INGREDIENTS

A scant pinch of saffron
3 cups milk
¼ tsp cardamom, ground
A pinch of salt
½ cup semolina (sooji)
3 tbsp honey
3 tbsp ghee (optional)
Pistachios chopped, for garnish

INSTRUCTIONS

Bring the saffron threads and milk to a boil and add the cardamom and salt. Lower the heat. In a steady stream, add the semolina, whisking continually until it is completely incorporated and there are no lumps. Lower the heat to its lowest setting. Cover and simmer for another 2–3 minutes. Once done, semolina will clump up within minutes. If you are not serving it immediately, add more milk or water to thin it out, whisking constantly. Swirl the honey and ghee in just before serving and garnish with chopped pistachios.

NOTES

Saffron adds incredible depth and richness to this simple breakfast. Ghee is optional but highly recommended at the finish. Add sliced banana or some other fruit in place of honey. Top with a mixture of granola or seeds and nuts of your choice.

Tomato Mint Raita

Serves 3–4

Preparation time: 20 minutes

INGREDIENTS

2 cups plain yoghurt

1 tsp ground cumin

1 tsp salt

2 tsp sugar

1 cup chopped tomatoes

¼ cup red onion, diced

1 tbsp mint, minced

3 tbsp olive oil

1 tsp mustard seeds

INSTRUCTIONS

Whisk the yoghurt into a large bowl. Season with salt, cumin and sugar. Chop the tomatoes into ½ inch pieces. Fold into yoghurt along with red onion and mint. Heat up the oil in a small saucepan and pop the mustard seeds. Fold this into the raita and serve. The raita can be kept in the fridge for up to 2 days. If you notice any water, separate from the yoghurt, you can simply drain it off before serving.

NOTES

Top with 1 tsp of lemon juice for added brightness. Substitute sugar with honey or ½ cup of mangoes. Add sunflower seeds for an extra crunch.

Turmeric Rice

Serves 4
Preparation time: 30 minutes–1 hour (for soaking)
Cooking time: 20 minutes

INGREDIENTS

1½ cups (250 g) basmati rice

3 tbsp ghee or oil

1 tsp mustard seeds

1 tsp turmeric

1 tsp salt

Nuts, dry fruit, seeds, herbs (optional, as toppings)

INSTRUCTIONS

Rinse the basmati rice in water twice. Soak for 30 minutes to one hour in 3 cups of water. Drain by pouring out most of the water. A little remaining water is okay. In a stockpot, heat the ghee until it is shimmering but not smoking. Add the mustard seeds. They will pop and sizzle. Almost immediately, add the drained rice, 2½ cups of water, turmeric, and salt. Bring the mixture to a boil, then cover and turn to low. Cook for another 5–7 minutes or until almost all of the water has been absorbed, then turn the heat off. Let the rice rest for 10–15 minutes and then serve.

NOTES

Turmeric adds a golden colour and earthy taste to the long-grain basmati rice. Pop the mustard seeds in ghee for maximum flavour. Add one cup of frozen or fresh peas to the rice 2–3 minutes before it is done. Add orange zest from 2 oranges when adding rice and water to the stockpot. Substitute cumin for mustard seeds. Add a whole stick of cinnamon for added fragrance.

Vegetable Dal Soup

Serves 4
Preparation time: 2–3 hours (for soaking)
Cooking time: 30 minutes

INGREDIENTS

1 cup toor dal
½ tsp turmeric
1 tsp grated unpeeled ginger
3–4 cloves, crushed
1 stick of cinnamon
3–4 tbsp olive oil or ghee
1 tsp black mustard seeds
½ cup minced green onion
1 serrano pepper, minced
3 cups of green beans, trimmed and cut into 1-inch pieces
1 cup tomatoes, chopped
½ cup peanuts

1 tbsp jaggery

2 tsp salt

Juice from half a lemon

½ cup chopped fresh coriander

INSTRUCTIONS

Rinse the lentils 2–3 times and soak for 2–3 hours. Drain, combine with 5 cups of water in a stockpot, and bring to a boil. Discard the scum that may arise. Add the turmeric, ginger, cloves, and cinnamon. Turn the heat down, cover the pot, and simmer for an hour or more. The lentils should be soft and completely dissolved. In a separate frying pan, heat the olive oil. When it is just shy of smoking, add the mustard seeds and let them pop and sizzle. Almost immediately, add the green onion, serrano pepper, and green beans and cook on high heat until they have a little bit of colour. Add tomatoes, peanuts, jaggery, and salt and continue cooking for another 2–3 minutes. Transfer this mixture to the dal and continue simmering for another 10 minutes. If the dal appears too thick, add half a cup of water. Stir the lemon juice and coriander into the soup and serve.

NOTES

Toor dal, a humble yet deeply delicious flat yellow pigeon pea lentil, is nutritiously dense, and high in fibre, complex carbohydrates, folic acid, and protein. It makes the base for the delicious South Indian sambhar, and while this soup is a lot simpler version of that, it works as a vehicle for seasonal vegetables—so feel free to adapt based on what is at hand. If you must replace the toor dal, use the yellow moong or the orange lentil. Replace green beans with carrots, cauliflower or any seasonal vegetables.

Recipes to Soothe Your System

	Weight Loss	Mouth Sores/ Dry Mouth	Diarrhoea	Constipation	Nausea/ Vomiting
• Green Gram Soup		X			X
• Yellow Pumpkin Soup		X			X
• Mulligatawny Soup		X			
• Ginger Tea					X
• Honey-Lime Soda		X	X	X	X
• Tomato Chutney		X			
• Cucumber Raita	X	X	X		X
• Tomato Mint Raita	X	X	X		X
• Ginger Smoothie	X	X	X		X
• Unripe and Ripe Mango Smoothie	X	X			X
• Vegetable Dal Soup		X			X

	Weight Loss	Mouth Sores/ Dry Mouth	Diarrhoea	Constipation	Nausea/ Vomiting
• Date and Fig Smoothie	X	X			
• Sweet Corn Smoothie	X	X			
• Papaya/ Mango and Honey Smoothie	X	X		X	
• Green Papaya Salad					
• Chana with Lime and Garlic	X				
• Sabudana Khichdi	X				X
• Rice Undas	X		X		X
• Semiya Idli	X		X		X
• Kanda Poha	X				
• Olan	X				
• Chicken Stew	X	X			X
• Green Moong Pancake	X				

	Weight Loss	Mouth Sores/ Dry Mouth	Diarrhoea	Constipation	Nausea/ Vomiting
• Sweet and Sour Pumpkin Bharta	X				
• Pressed Rice with Vegetables, Eggs and Cottage Cheese	X				
• Saffron Halwa	X	X			
• Honey Laced 'Pongal'	X	X			X
• Chickpea Chilla w/ Avocado Masala	X				
• Cheese Toast	X				
• Chicken Pakora with Mint Chutney	X				
• Turmeric Rice	X	X	X		

	Weight Loss	Mouth Sores/ Dry Mouth	Diarrhoea	Constipation	Nausea/ Vomiting
• Khichdi	X	X	X		X
• Fruit custard	X			X	
• Chikoo Kheer	X			X	
• Chicken Stir-fry	X				
• Parijat Kalakand	X				
• Fruit Chaat	X			X	

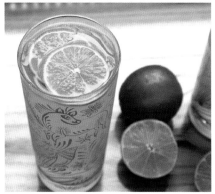

Honey Lime Soda
(p. 134)

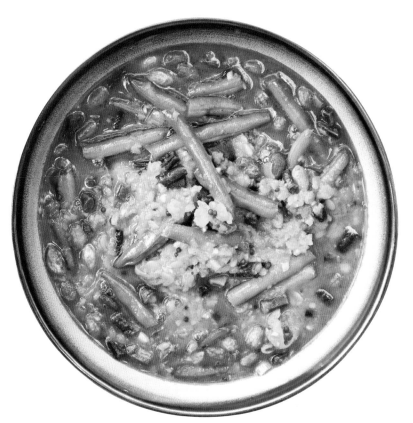

Vegetable Dal Soup
(p. 139)

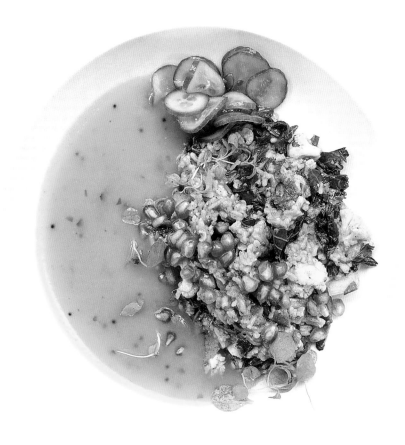

Khichdi
(p. 135)

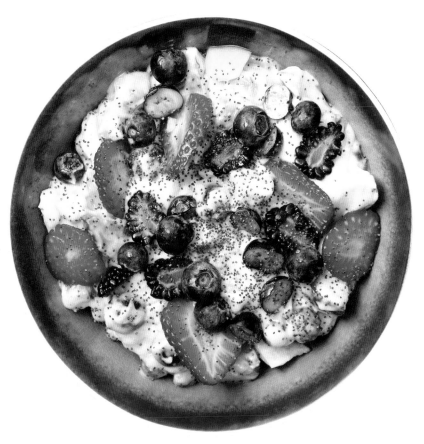

Fruit Custard
(p. 132)

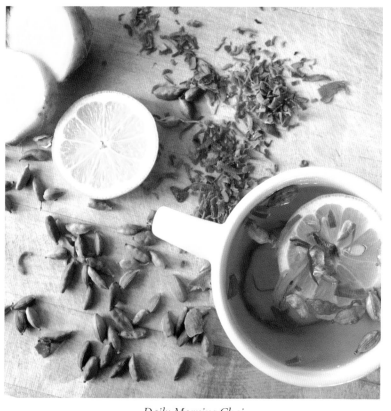

Daily Morning Chai
(p. 125)

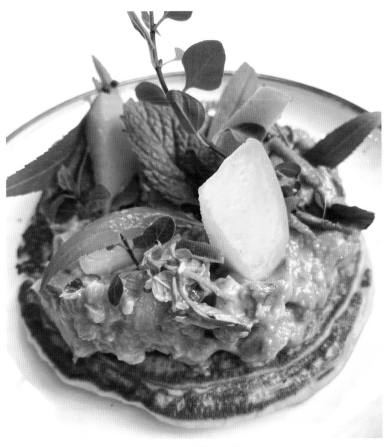

Chickpea Chilla with
Avocado Masala
(p. 128)

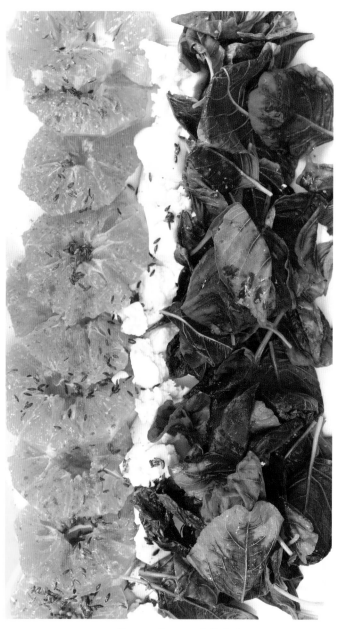

Orange Amaranth Salad
(p. 166)

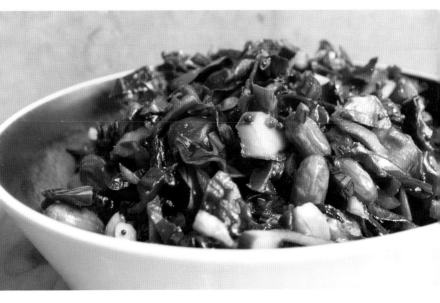

Jain Cabbage Salad
(p. 164)

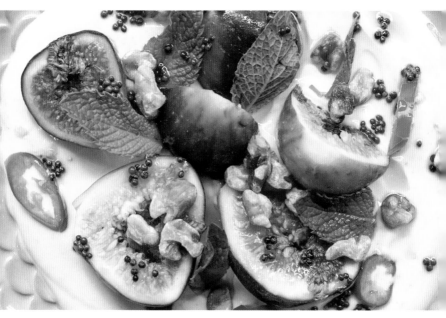

Fig Yoghurt Salad
(p. 163)

SECTION III

Surviving Cancer

In every end, there is also a beginning.
—ANONYMOUS

1

Caring for Your Body After Treatment

Krishan Kalra noticed a change when he woke up one morning. He had a tiny spot of blood on his night shirt that initially used to appear weekly, but its frequency changed to almost daily. He had a busy schedule as he had just taken over as the Secretary General of the PhD Chamber in New Delhi. He was not overly concerned, but called his general practitioner who, alarmed by his symptoms, got him to come in the same day. A mammogram, ultrasound, and biopsy later, his worst fears were confirmed when his doctor looked at his slides and uttered the life-altering words: 'This does not look good.'

Male breast cancer is not a myth; it is very much a reality. In the US and UK, male breast cancer accounts for 0.5 per cent to 1 per cent of total cases. It is a common misconception that as men do not have breasts, they cannot get breast cancer. The fact is that both men and women have breast tissue. The difference is that women possess hormones that lead to further development of this tissue, which is not the case in men. However, this tissue in men can give rise to cancer in a similar fashion like it does with women. It commonly presents itself as a firm and painless lump in the breast, but is ignored by most men. Even though a lot still needs to be done for breast cancer awareness in women, at least there is general knowledge that a lump in the breast can be cancerous. This is not the case as far as men are concerned. In a majority of cases, a delay in diagnosis lessens the chance of cure—the disease is already too advanced. The treatment for male breast cancer is similar to that for women—incorporating surgery, radiation, and chemotherapy. Fortunately for Mr Kalra his cancer was diagnosed early and he underwent surgery followed by anti-hormonal therapy. On the advice of his physicians, he modified his diet and incorporated regular exercise into his routine. The end of cancer therapy is truly a new beginning, marking the shift from patient to survivor. This is a critical stage, as individuals who have been diagnosed with cancer are at a significantly higher risk of developing new cancer.[155] They also can be at increased risk of chronic diseases such as bone loss, diabetes, and heart disease.[156]

Exercise: Just Do It

Observational studies in survivors of breast, colorectal, and prostate cancers demonstrated that physically active cancer survivors had improved survival compared to those who were inactive. Exercise has also demonstrated to improve fatigue, self-esteem, depression, and overall happiness and quality of life in survivors of cancer. A meta-analysis of 12,108 patients with breast cancer demonstrated that post-diagnosis physical activity reduced breast cancer deaths by 34 per cent and disease recurrence by 24 per cent.[157] Patients with prostate cancer are frequently treated with androgen blocker therapy to decrease testosterone, which can result in muscle wasting and decreased bone mass. Fifty-seven patients with prostate cancer undergoing therapy were randomly assigned to a programme of resistance and aerobic exercise or usual care for 12 weeks. Participants undertook combined progressive resistance and aerobic training twice a week for 12 weeks. The resistance exercises included chest press, seated row, shoulder press, triceps extension, leg press, leg extension, and leg curl, with abdominal crunches also performed. The sessions started and concluded with general flexibility exercises. The aerobic component of the training program included 15 to 20 minutes of cardiovascular exercises (cycling and walking/jogging) at 65 per cent to 80 per cent maximum heart rate. The patients who were exposed to aerobic exercise had significantly improved muscle mass, strength, physical function, and balance compared with normal care.[158]

This is not to say that everyone should get on a treadmill immediately. After discussing with your healthcare team, start with what is feasible. You can start with 10 minutes of light exercise daily and slowly work your way up. The doctor's involvement in this process is vital as it has been demonstrated that physician advice can be a powerful force in facilitating preventative health behaviours. In a study, breast cancer survivors were randomly assigned to receive a doctor's exercise recommendation only, an exercise recommendation and referral to an exercise specialist, or a standard follow-up. The primary outcome was self-reported total exercise at five weeks after the initial consultation. The researchers found that the doctor's recommendation led to a significant increase in exercise behaviour in patients, particularly if it was recalled one week after the recommendation.[159]

Guidelines for survivors for aerobic physical activity recommend that adults aged 18 to 64 years should engage in at least 150 minutes per week of moderate intensity (for example, walking briskly, playing doubles tennis) or 75 minutes per week of vigorous intensity aerobic physical activity (race walking, jogging, or running), or an equivalent combination of moderate and vigorous intensity aerobic physical activity. They also recommend that some exercise is better than none. In addition, adults should do muscle-strengthening activities involving all major muscle groups at least two days per week.[160] Adults older than 65 years of age should still try to incorporate physical exercise, as tolerated, and avoid long periods of inactivity. The most critical component of being physically active is the support structure as only 20–30 per cent of cancer survivors will get active after their therapy has ended.[161] This underscores the importance of support groups, supervised exercise, counselling, and follow-up to encourage physical activity in survivors.

Tobacco: Just DON'T Do It

Patients frequently ask me: 'Doc, I already have cancer. How does it matter if I continue to smoke?' The answer is simple: you have been given a new lease on life, don't burn it by relapsing. Also, if you continue to smoke during treatment, it can make therapy harder and can prolong your recovery. A study examined the influence of cigarette smoking on side effects among 947 cancer patients during and six months following cancer treatment. They found that smokers reported significantly higher levels of symptom burden (problems with concentration, skin, sleep, weight loss, and depression). This higher symptom burden can lead to treatment interference, dose delays, and reductions or early stopping of therapy. In addition, the decrease in the symptom burden from the end of treatment to the six-month follow-up was significantly less for smokers than for non-smokers. Smokers also reported higher rates of severe side effects like acute fatigue, hair loss, concentration problems, hot flashes, skin problems, sleep problems, and depression six months after treatment.[162]

Smoking during therapy can also accelerate breakdown of some cancer therapies, leading to insufficient levels of the cancer therapy in blood. For example, erlotinib, a drug frequently used for lung cancer patients exhibited rapid clearance in smokers, requiring a higher dose to reach equal exposure compared with non-smokers: so more drug was required for the same effect.[163]

Quitting smoking can decrease your risk of recurrence (original cancer coming back) and also your risk of a second primary cancer (completely new and separate cancer which is unrelated to the original cancer). For example, if a patient had lung cancer and continues to smoke, they can end up with a second primary like cancer of the head and neck. A study followed lung cancer survivors and found an increased risk of cancer recurrence with patients who continued smoking. In fact, every additional pack a patient smoked per year increased the risk of having lung cancer again by 1 per cent.[164]

Similarly, a study in patients with breast cancer demonstrated a higher risk of death among women who continued smoking after diagnosis compared with patients who never smoked. The study authors concluded that 'Smoking negatively impacts long-term survival after breast cancer. Post-diagnosis cessation of smoking may reduce the risk of all-cause mortality. Breast cancer survivors may benefit from aggressive smoking cessation programs starting as early as the time of diagnosis.'[165] It is well known that the best time to quit is right after diagnosis. In fact, quitting smoking doesn't just decrease your risk of the cancer coming back, it increases your survival overall. And once you quit, your body begins to heal in a matter of a few minutes and the benefits continue throughout your life.[166]

All You Need is Love (and a Support System)

Survivors also struggle with weight management as some patients can end up gaining weight during chemotherapy. This has been reported for a number of cancers including breast and prostate. An analyses of non-smoking breast cancer survivors within the Nurses' Health Study reported that women who increased their BMI by 0.5 to 2 units were found to have a 40 per cent greater chance of recurrence (disease coming back), and those who gained more than 2 BMI units had a 53 per cent greater chance of recurrence compared with those who did not gain more than 0.5 BMI units. These associations with weight were stronger in premenopausal than in postmenopausal women.[167] Chemotherapy can cause temporary or permanent early menopause in women with breast cancer, resulting in physiological changes and subsequent weight gain. In addition, the shock of a cancer diagnosis, the stress of the change in lifestyle, steroids during chemotherapy, financial stress, and decreased physical activity on account of fatigue, all may contribute to weight gain. This is concerning as being overweight and obese are associated with an increased risk of cancer recurrence and impacts survival after cancer has gone into remission.

To help with weight loss, active intervention with lots of support is the secret. The Exercise and Nutrition to Enhance Recovery and Good Health for You (ENERGY) trial randomized 692 overweight/obese women (BMI of 25 to 45 kg/m^2) who were, on

average, two years since primary treatment for breast cancer post-
therapy, and assigned to active intervention or control intervention,
and observed for two years.[168]

The intervention began with an intensive phase that consisted
of four months of weekly one-hour group sessions followed by
every other week for two months, and then the groups met monthly
for the remainder of the first year. The strategies and guidance
discussed in the group sessions were reinforced by a telephone
call and/or by email. The goal of dietary guidance was to promote
a reduction in energy intake, aiming for a deficit of 500 to 1,000
kcal a day relative to expenditure. The physical activity goal was
an average of at least 60 minutes per day of purposeful exercise at
a moderate level of intensity. They also received specially tailored
print newsletters about physical activity, dietary intake, and weight;
and were provided guidance for overcoming barriers to increase
physical activity and regulate dietary intake.

Control group participants were provided weight management
resources and materials which existed in the public domain. An
individualized diet counselling session was provided at baseline and
at six months, and current physical activity recommendations (at
least 30 minutes per day) were advised. Control group participants
also received monthly telephone calls and/or emails from the study
coordinator and were invited to attend optional informational
seminars on aspects of healthy living other than weight control
every other month during the first year.

The researchers found that at 12 months, mean weight loss
was significantly better in the intervention group—6.0 per cent
versus 1.5 per cent in the control group. Interestingly, the weight
loss intervention was more effective among women older than 55
years than among younger women.

Another trial, the Women's Intervention Nutrition Study (WINS), tested the effect of a dietary intervention to reduce fat intake in 2,437 women with resected breast cancer. They found that a low-fat diet that resulted in a 6-pound weight loss corresponded with a reduction in the risk of the cancer recurring amongst postmenopausal breast cancer survivors (especially those with tumors that were hormone negative).[169] Thus, weight loss constitutes an important piece of the survivorship puzzle and is recommended that during, and more importantly after the therapy, survivors should strive to maintain a BMI between 18.5 kg/m^2 and 25 kg/m^2.[170]

Interestingly, in patients with breast cancer, weight gain seems to be selective and more due to accumulation of adipose tissue (fat) with loss of lean body mass (good muscle mass).[171] Just losing weight is not good enough: it is also important to build lean muscle mass. This can be achieved through exercise, especially resistance training. While a majority of survivors struggle with weight gain, patients with tumors of the head and neck maybe malnourished from treatment and require interventions to attain a healthy weight.

Back to Life, Back to Reality

Cancer changes everything. It makes one take a pause and re-evaluate life. When you are going through active therapy, the adrenaline is cruising through your body and all your energy is focused on getting to the end of therapy. Resolves are made and diets changed. It can be an emotional roller-coaster when you are in the midst of therapy. However, it is important to be aware of the time when therapy ends and the adrenaline rush dissipates. It is at this crucial juncture that diet and exercise commitments have to transform into a lifestyle change. Re-evaluate your diet and identify areas where changes can be made. Researchers evaluated dietary patterns in 1,901 survivors with early-stage breast cancer. They found that women who followed a prudent dietary pattern (defined as a diet with high intake of fruits and vegetables and whole grains) had a 43 per cent reduction in overall risk of death as compared to those who had dietary patterns that have been characterized as Western (high intakes of meat, refined grains, and high-fat foods).[172]

Another observational study of patients with colorectal cancer who had undergone surgery and chemotherapy found that a diet characterized by higher intake of processed and red meat, fat, sugary desserts, and refined grains was associated with a higher rate of cancer recurrence and death.[173]

While studies looked at dietary patterns holistically, some studies have tried to look at specific components of diet. Two large studies in breast cancer tested the hypothesis of fat reduction in patients after therapy for breast cancer. The WINS study mentioned previously tested a low-fat diet in postmenopausal women with breast cancer. They reported an 18 per cent decrease in dietary fat intake and a mean weight loss of 6 pounds at 12 months in the intervention group that resulted in a 24 per cent decrease in new cases of breast cancer. However, it is hard to say if the improvement was on account of the reduced fat or the weight loss.[174] Another trial, the Women's Healthy Eating and Living (WHEL), tested a diet low in fat (with a goal of fat as 20 per cent of daily expenditure) in 3,000 women after therapy for breast cancer.[175] They reported a decrease in the fat intake from 31 per cent at enrollment to 26 per cent, but no decrease in the recurrence of breast cancer. One of the differences in the two studies was that in addition to reducing fat, women in the WINS study also lost weight, which as discussed earlier, could be a differentiating factor. Men with prostate cancer may also benefit from watching their cholesterol levels as they are at a greater risk of death due to heart disease.

When it comes to choices after the end of therapy, here are a few tips that can be of help in your post-cancer journey:

- A 'prudent' dietary pattern is one that predominantly involves fruits and vegetables, protein from sources like fish and white meat rather than red meat or processed foods, and carbohydrates from whole grains instead of polished grains.

- Try limiting consumption of red and processed meats, alcohol, and energy-dense or junk foods (potato chips, French fries, hot dogs)[176] and increase consumption of plant-based foods (vegetables, fruits, whole grains). ESPEN guidelines are similar in its recommendations to 'maintain a healthy weight (BMI 18.5-25 kg/m^2) and to maintain a healthy lifestyle, which includes being physically active and a diet based on vegetables, fruits and whole grains and low in saturated fat, red meat and alcohol.'

- It is increasingly clear that being overweight after therapy can be associated with poorer survival and a higher chance of cancer recurrence; hence, it is important to try and maintain a healthy weight after the end of therapy. Exercise and physical activity after diagnosis has been associated with a lower risk of disease recurrence and improved survival primarily in patients with breast, ovarian, prostate, and colorectal cancers. Exercise also improves the overall quality of life by improving fatigue, muscle strength and anxiety, and helps boost self-esteem.

Hence, in addition to modifying the diet, weight loss (if appropriate) and exercise can have a synergistic effect in improving survival and quality of life outcomes in survivors recovering from therapy.

Yes to Life

Cancer therapy is akin to a roller-coaster ride: lots of ups and downs, twists and turns. Expect the unexpected. But, there is light at the end of the tunnel for patients who are receiving therapy to improve their rate of recovery and all you are doing is looking at that moment. Once that exhilarating day comes, it is important not to get complacent and get ready for the marathon of survivorship after the sprint during therapy. One of my friends, a colleague and a cancer survivor himself, has put this perfectly: 'While I empathize with the way "scanxiety" (anxiety about scans) punctuates our equilibrium, I'm more familiar with the almost-mundane sense of inhabiting a broken body that you can't escape'.

After therapy is over, the adrenaline subsides and the mundane reality sets in—though it may look different than before your cancer was diagnosed—there are a number of fears the survivor can face. And there can be lingering effects, both physical and psychological. The protective cocoon that surrounds you during therapy is lost with less frequent visits to the doctor and nurse. Friends and family may also take a step back. The fear of recurrence is common in cancer survivors who say that the thought of recurrence is still omnipresent, with each check-up bringing anxiety with it. With time, some of these fears may dissipate, but it is rare for them to go away altogether. You can also feel added stress, depression, and loneliness as it may be hard to relate to friends and family members who might mean well, but have not been in your shoes. At this stage, it is important to have open and frank discussions with your healthcare team, friends and family, and support groups, where you will meet people who have been through similar experiences.

After overcoming her cancer for the second time, Anjali's attitude changed and she tries to take things one day at a time. She helps women who are going through cancer diagnosis and therapy. Mr Kalra started volunteering with various cancer organizations and started living by the motto: Don't worry about tomorrow. Before she was diagnosed, Mrs Menon was working on getting permission to set up a library. The same year she was diagnosed, she received permission and worked with her friends to get the library up and running. It has not been easy, her diet and taste buds have changed, but she has adjusted. She is a phenomenal cook and shares her delectable recipes with cancer patients. Her advice: 'Be aware, not scared; when it comes to therapy. Don't waffle—take a decision, go with it, and don't look back. Educate yourself, keep your friends and family close, and most importantly, keep yourself busy.' And that's exactly what Shruti and Neeti did. Neeti founded Yes to Life a non-governmental organization (NGO), and later Shruti joined as an honorary vice-president. This NGO helps other young survivors connect to a support group which provides a positive outlook, faith, and strength to manage the phases of diagnosis, treatment, and after-treatment successfully. In addition, they run cancer-screening camps and provide support (emotional, financial and for rehabilitation) for needy patients. They also help patients diagnosed with cancer in the age group of 20–50 years deal with issues relating to communicating the diagnosis with children and those relating to fertility, body image, career, intimacy, etc.

Recovery from cancer therapy is truly about healing your body, mind and soul. To help kick-start this next chapter in your life, we have included recipes that you can make together with your support group. Time is a great healer, and grit, determination and help of family and friends can make it all possible. We wish you the best of luck in your nutrition and health journey for the next phase of your life. The future, friends is truly bright!!

Recipes

CONTRIBUTED BY SWATI PANT AND ANITA JAISINGHANIA

Cucumber and Peanut Salad

Serves 2

Preparation time: 10 minutes

INGREDIENTS

2 large or 3 medium cucumbers
¼ cup roasted peanuts
¼ cup fresh grated coconut (optional)
1 tbsp fresh coriander leaves, chopped
2–3 tsp lime juice
Pink salt to taste

INSTRUCTIONS

Peel the cucumber and chop into small pieces. Crush the peanuts into chunky pieces. Add the chopped coriander and coconut. Mix all the ingredients together with lime juice. Season right before serving.

NOTES

This salad can also be made with a mix of cucumber and bell peppers or only with capsicum also.

Cottage Cheese (Paneer) and Grape Salad

Serves 2

Preparation time: 10 minutes

INGREDIENTS

150 gm fresh paneer (home-made or store bought)
2 small bunches of grapes (green/ red/ black or a mix of all)

½ tsp cumin powder, roasted

¾ tsp black fruit chaat masala (optional)

Rock salt to taste (if your fruit chaat masala is unsalted)

1 small lime

INSTRUCTIONS

Cut the paneer into cubes. Halve the grapes and mix with the paneer cubes. Now add the spices and toss together with the juice of one lime. Adjust the seasoning. Chill for 10 minutes before serving.

NOTES

The above salad can also be made with watermelon. Double the quantity of watermelon to paneer and garnish with fresh chopped mint.

Whole Red Lentils Salad
(Sabut Masoor Dal)

Serves 2-3

Preparation time: 30 minutes (for soaking the dal)

Cooking time: 20 minutes

INGREDIENTS

1 cup sabut masoor dal

½ cup pomegranate seeds

1 cucumber

½ cup baby spinach leaves (optional)

2 tbsp almonds, toasted and sliced

2 tsp olive oil (optional)

Juice of 1 lemon

Rock Salt

Pepper

INSTRUCTIONS

Wash and soak the masoor dal for 30 minutes. Drain and change the water. Boil the dal in a pressure cooker until cooked but not mushy. Skin and chop the cucumber into small pieces. Once the daal is cooled, tip into a bowl and add cucumber, pomegranate, and baby spinach leaves, if using. Mix olive oil, lemon juice, salt, and pepper and pour the dressing over the salad. Garnish with sliced almonds. Cool and enjoy.

NOTES

You could add fresh grated coconut as a garnish if you like.

Fig Yoghurt Salad

Serves 3

Preparation time: 15 minutes + overnight for yoghurt

INGREDIENTS

8–10 fresh figs

1 cup yoghurt

A scant pinch of saffron

¼ tsp cumin

2 pinches of salt

2 tbsp mustard oil

½ tsp mustard seeds

½ small green chilli, minced

10–12 mint leaves

2 tbsp walnuts

INSTRUCTIONS

Stir the yoghurt with the saffron, ground cumin, and salt and set it aside, preferably overnight. Slice the figs in half and generously sprinkle with salt. Chill until ready to serve. Just before serving, smear the yoghurt onto a plate. Arrange the figs on top and scatter the minced green chilli around. Heat up the mustard oil and pop the mustard seeds. Spoon this over the figs and yoghurt. Tuck the mint leaves and walnuts in and around the figs.

NOTES

This salad makes a great first course. The burn of the mustard oil plays beautifully with the cool creaminess of the saffron yogurt and the rich, sweet figs. The saffron needs time to infuse into the yoghurt, so it is best made the day before or at least a few hours before.

Jain Cabbage Salad

Serves 3–4

Preparation time: 15 minutes

INGREDIENTS

3 tbsp peanut oil

A pinch of asafoetida

8–10 curry leaves (kadi patta), chopped

1 tsp mustard seeds

½ head of a small purple cabbage (approximately 3 cups, 220 g)

1 serrano pepper, sliced

Juice from one lemon

2 tbsp mint leaves, chopped

1 cup toasted peanuts, whole

1 tsp salt

INSTRUCTIONS

Heat the sesame oil in a skillet and pop the asafoetida, curry leaves, and mustard seeds. Add the sliced cabbage and serrano peppers. Cook on high heat until they are just wilted, 2–3 minutes at the most. Turn the heat off and transfer the cabbage to a bowl. Stir in the lemon juice, mint leaves, peanuts, and salt.

NOTES

Instead of asafoetida, use 1 tsp minced garlic. Try cumin seeds instead of mustard seeds.

Masala Boiled Egg Salad

Serves 4–5

Cooking time: 30 minutes

INGREDIENTS

4 fresh eggs

2 cups of salad greens (spinach or lettuce)

1 medium tomato, cut into 1 inch chunks

½ tsp salt

A pinch of red chilli powder

2 tbsp olive oil

1 tsp cumin seeds

½ cup of diced red onion

1 tsp green chilli, minced
Juice from half a lemon
A pinch of salt

INSTRUCTIONS

Bring the eggs to a boil and cook for 8–10 minutes. Turn off the heat and let the eggs rest in warm water for 15–20 minutes. Remove shell and slice into 4 pieces. On a shallow serving bowl, spread the salad greens and scatter the tomato over it. Next, spread the sliced eggs on the greens. Sprinkle salt and chilli powder over the entire mixture. Heat up the olive oil and pop the cumin seeds. Add the diced red onion and green chilli and cook on medium heat for 3–4 minutes or until the onion are translucent. Drizzle over the salad greens, add the lemon juice and additional salt to taste. Toss and serve.

NOTES

This recipe circumvents the boiled egg taste and gives it a fragrant ginger flavour. Feel free to add other vegetables like cucumber or radish to the salad.

Orange Amaranth Salad
(Rajgira)

Serves 3–4 servings
Preparation time: 30 min

INGREDIENTS

4–5 cups of amaranth leaves
Juice from one lemon
3 oranges
A pinch of chilli powder
150 gm goat cheese or paneer

2 tbsp olive oil

1 tsp cumin seeds

Salt to taste

INSTRUCTIONS

Toss the amaranth leaves with lemon and salt and refrigerate until ready to use. Peel the 3 oranges and slice them horizontally (about ½ inch thick) and lay them on a serving plate. Sprinkle the orange slices with a pinch of salt and chilli powder. Heat the olive oil until just shy of smoking and add the cumin seeds. Within seconds, the seeds will pop and sizzle. Turn the heat off and drizzle the hot oil over the sliced tangerines. Crumble or cut the cheese into pieces and place it next to the orange slices. Spread the marinated amaranth leaves next to the cheese and serve.

NOTES

Replace the cumin seeds with coriander seeds. Be careful when popping seeds to ensure they don't burn or the salad will turn bitter. The salad can be prepared ahead of time and kept refrigerated for up to 6 hours. Even if the amaranth leaves wilt, they still taste really good.

Tomato Salad

Serves 3

Preparation time: 10 minutes

INGREDIENTS

2–3 large tomatoes, cut into thick slices

1 firm but ripe mango, chopped

¼ tsp salt

¼ tsp ground cumin

¼ tsp chilli powder

3 tbsp mustard oil

½ tsp coriander seeds

3 tbsp pistachios, chopped

A few sprigs of coriander leaves

INSTRUCTIONS

Lay the tomatoes on a serving platter. Scatter the mango on top. Sprinkle with salt, ground cumin, and chilli powder. Heat the mustard oil and pop the coriander seeds. Drizzle on the tomatoes and mangoes. Garnish with chopped pistachios and coriander leaves. This salad is good on its own and also makes an good side dish for tandoori or roasted meats.

NOTES

Add mild cheese like paneer or mozzarella. Spread on top of warm toast for a tasty starter or toss with greens to make a salad.

Acknowledgements

I have many people to thank for helping me in life and in the journey of this book. First and foremost, I wanted to thank my wife, Srishti Mehta, without whose love and support this book would have been impossible to finish.

To my daughters, Anya and Shreya who bring immense joy in my life.

To my father, Dr (Col.) C.S. Pant, VSM, who is my inspiration. He is an amazing father, empathetic physician and human being who has dedicated his life to helping people. To my mother, Geeta Pant, who has been our family rock and who taught us the value of hard work and honesty.

To my grandmother (my Naani Maa), who taught me never to give up regardless of the challenges. My in-laws, Siddhartha and Vanita Mehta, for their input on the book and more importantly, for allowing me to marry their daughter. My sister Swati Pant, who has helped me at every turn in life, contributed to recipes in the book and is an amazing chef. Thank you Vineet (my brother-in-law) for entertaining Anya and Shreya during their spring break, affording me time to get the book done.

A big thanks to Anita Jaisinghania, chef extraordinaire, who was kind enough to share her recipes and helped provide creative input including photographs of her recipes. Pushpesh Pant, who has an encyclopedic knowledge of Indian foods and is very generous in sharing his knowledge.

To the amazing survivors and spouses who opened up to me about their cancer journey: Mrs Prasanna Menon, Neeti Leekha, Shruti Sharma, Anjali Sapra, Mr Krishan Kalra, Pragya and IP Tewari. To all of you, I am deeply indebted.

I wanted to thank my publishers HarperCollins India—Debasri Rakshit, my commissioning editor who helped kick start the book, Shreya Punj for helping shape the book during the 'slog years', Sonal Nerurkar and Diya Kar who helped take it across the finish line. My *Living it Up* friends Vaishali Sood and Amrita Tripathi, my sounding boards who gave me great, honest feedback from the content to the naming of the book. A special thank you to Amrita who, along with being amazingly talented, is one of the nicest people I know and was very generous with her time. I think it is fair to say that without her invaluable help and support this book would never have been possible.

This book required extensive background research and I very much appreciate Dr George and Sukanya for their help.

Dr Goldy C George earned a PhD in Nutritional Sciences from the University of Texas at Austin and previously a Master's degree in Foods and Nutrition from the University of Madras in Chennai, India. She is currently an Assistant Professor in the Department of Symptom Research at The University of Texas M.D. Anderson Cancer Center, Houston, TX, USA. Her research interests include the role of diet in affecting cancer-related clinical outcomes and symptomatic burden in patients with cancer and in cancer survivors. Her contributions to this book included research and writing on global dietary recommendations to prevent or control cancer, and the scientific basis of these recommendations.

Sukanya Sharma works as a writer in Mumbai with various publications. A history graduate to advertising professional to mental health advocate, she is now working on her project The Caravan Cult to build educational programmes on sustainability through a travel module.

Most importantly, I wanted to thank my patients and their caregivers who inspired me to write this book. They teach me something every day and help me appreciate life on a daily basis. My heartfelt and humble thanks.

Notes and References

1. Mallath, Mohandas K. et al. 'The growing burden of cancer in India: epidemiology and social context', *The Lancet Oncology*, vol. 15, no. 6, 2014.

2. Goodwin, C. J., *Research In Psychology: Methods and Design*, 7th Edition, Hoboken: Wiley, 2012.

3. Inoue-Choi Maki, Oppeneer Sarah J. and Robien Kim, 'Reality Check: There is No Such Thing as a Miracle Food, Nutrition and Cancer', https://doi.org/10.1080/01635581.2013.748921, 65:2, 165-168, 2013.

4. Bagri, Neha T., 'A growing taste for US fast food in India', CNBC, https://www.cnbc.com/2014/01/08/a-growing-taste-for-us-fast-food-in-india.html [accessed: 20 July 2020].

5. Singh, P. N. et al., 'Global epidemiology of obesity, vegetarian dietary patterns, and noncommunicable disease in Asian Indians', *The American Journal of Clinical Nutrition*, vol. 100 Suppl 1,1, 2014, pp. 359S–64S.

6. Bhushan, Chandra, Taneja, Sonam and Khurana, Amit, 'Burden of Packaged Food on Schoolchildren: Based on the CSE Survey "Know Your Diet",' Centre for Science and

Environment, New Delhi 2017, https://rb.gy/n3xyg3 [accessed: 5 November 2020].

7.   Singh, P. N. et al., 'Global epidemiology of obesity, vegetarian dietary patterns, and noncommunicable disease in Asian Indians', *The American Journal of Clinical Nutrition*, vol. 100 Suppl 1,1, 2014, pp. 359S–64S.

8.   Arora N.K. et al., 'Whole-of-society monitoring framework for sugar, salt, and fat consumption and noncommunicable diseases in India', *Annals of the New York Academy of Sciences*, vol. 133, no. 1, December 2014, pp. 157–73.

9.   Prentice, R. L. et al., 'Regression calibration in nutritional epidemiology: example of fat density and total energy in relationship to postmenopausal breast cancer', *American Journal of Epidemiology*, vol. 178, no. 11, 2013, pp.1663–72.

10.   Albuquerque, R. C., Baltar, V. T., Marchioni, D. M., 'Breast cancer and dietary patterns: a systematic review', *Nutrition Review*, vol. 72, no. 1, 2014, pp. 1–17.

11.   Singh et al., 'Global epistemology of obesity, vegetarian dietary patterns, and noncommunicable disease in Asian Indians'.

12.   Nebehay, S., 'Smoking down, but tobacco use still a major cause of death, disease – WHO', *Reuters*, 31 May 2018, https://www.reuters.com/article/us-health-smoking/smoking-down-but-tobacco-use-still-a-major-cause-of-death-disease-who-idUSKCN1IV2W2 [accessed: 29 July 2020].

13.   'Prevalence of tobacco smoking', World Health Organization, 2016, http://gamapserver.who.int/gho/interactive_charts/tobacco/use/atlas.html [accessed: 29 July 2020].

14.   Ibid.

15.   Gupta, P. C. et al. (eds.), 'Smokeless Tobacco and Public Health in India', New Delhi: Ministry of Health and Family Welfare, Government of India, 2018.

16.   National Cancer Institute, www.cancer.gov [accessed: 29 July 2020]

17.   Centers for Disease CaP et al., 'How Tobacco Smoke Causes Disease: The Biology and Behavioral Basis for Smoking-Attributable Disease: A Report of the Surgeon General', Atlanta: Centers for Disease Control and Prevention, 2010 and World Health Organization, 'Tobacco Control: Reversal of Risk after Quitting Smoking', IARC Handbooks of Cancer Prevention, 2007, p. 341.

18.   Mayne, S. T., Playdon, M. C., and Rock, C. L., 'Diet, nutrition, and cancer: Past, present and future', *Nature Reviews, Clinical Oncology*, vol. 13, no. 8, 2016, pp. 504–15.

19.   Ibid.

20.   Ibid.

21.   Ibid.

22.   Sen, C. T., *Food Culture in India*, Westport: Greenwood Press, 2004.

23.   Singh, P. N. et al., 'Global epidemiology of obesity, vegetarian dietary patterns, and noncommunicable disease in Asian Indians'.

24.   Gopalan, C., Sastri, B. V. and Balasubramanian, S. C., *Nutritive Value of Indian Foods*. Revised and updated by Rao, Narasinga B.S., Deosthale, Y. G., and Pant, K. C., Hyderabad: National Institue of Nutrition, 1971, 1989, 2009.

25.   Dixit, A. A. et al., 'Incorporation of whole, ancient grains into a modern Asian Indian diet to reduce the burden of chronic disease', *Nutrition Reviews*, vol. 69, no. 8, 2011, pp. 479–88.

26.   Radhika, G. et al, 'Refined grain consumption and the metabolic syndrome in urban Asian Indians' (Chennai Urban Rural Epidemiology Study 57), *Metabolism: Clinical and Experimental*, vol. 58, 2009, pp. 675–81.

27. Sun, Q. et al., 'White rice, brown rice, and risk of type 2 diabetes in US men and women', *Archives of Internal Medicine*, vol. 170, no. 11, 2010, pp. 961–9.

28. Devi, P. B. et al., 'Health benefits of finger millet (Eleusine coracana L.) polyphenols and dietary fiber: a review', *Journal of Food Science an Technology*, vol. 51, no. 6, 2014, pp. 1021–40.

29. Ibid.

30. Ibid.

31. Ibid.

32. Ibid.

33. Ibid.

34. Cardoso, L. de Morais et al., 'Sorghum (Sorghum bicolor L.): Nutrients, bioactive compounds, and potential impact on human health', *Critical Reviews in Food Science and Nutrition*, vol. 57, no. 2, 2017, pp. 372–90.

35. Ibid.

36. Ibid.

37. Vasant, R. A., et al., 'Physiological role of a multigrain diet in metabolic regulations of lipid and antioxidant profiles in hypercholesteremic rats: multigrain diet in hyperlipemia', *Journal of Pharmacopuncture*, vol. 17, no. 2, 2014, pp. 34–40.

38. Shukla, K., et al., 'Glycaemic response to maize, bajra and barley', *Indian Journal of Physiology and Pharmacology*, vol. 35, no. 4, 1991, pp. 249–54.

39. Kumar, S. et al., 'Perceptions about varieties of brown rice: a qualitative study from southern India', *Journal of the American Dietic Association*, vol. 111, no. 10, 2011, pp. 1517–22.

40. Sen, C. T., *Food Culture in India*.

41. Al-Zalabani, A. H. and Stewart, K. F., Modifiable risk factors for the prevention of bladder cancer: a systematic review of meta-analyses', *European Journal of Epidermology*, vol. 31, no. 99, 2016, pp. 811–51.

42. Aune, D. et al., 'Fruit and vegetable intake and the risk of cardiovascular disease, total cancer and all-cause mortality-a systematic review and dose-response meta-analysis of prospective studies', *International Journal of Epidemiology*, vol. 46, no. 3, 2017, pp. 1029–56.

43. Bradbury K. E., Appleby, P. N. and Key, T. J., 'Fruit, vegetable, and fiber intake in relation to cancer risk: findings from the European Prospective Investigation into Cancer and Nutrition (EPIC)', *American Journal of Clinical Nutrition*, vol. 100, suppl. 1, 2014, pp. 394s–98s.

44. 'Dietary Guidelines for Indians: A Manual,' National Institute of Nutrition, Indian Council of Medical Research, 2011, https://www.nin.res.in/downloads/DietaryGuidelinesforNINwebsite.pdf

45. Devi P. B. et al., 'Health benefits of finger millet'.

46. Kumar, S. et al, 'Perceptions about varieties of brown rice'.

47. Ibid.

48. Bradbury, K. E., Appleby, P. N. and Key, T. J., 'Fruit, vegetable, and fiber intake in relation to cancer risk'.

49. Reynolds, A. et al., 'Carbohydrate quality and human health: a series of systematic reviews and meta-analyses', *The Lancet*, vol. 393, 2019, pp. 434–45.

50. Mintel Press Team, 'Indonesia and India among the world's fastest growing processed food retail markets', *Mintel Press Office*, 24 April 2017.

51. Norat, T, et al., 'European Code against Cancer 4th edition: Diet and cancer'. *Cancer Epidemiology*, vol. 39, suppl 1, 2015, pp. S56–66.

52. Helmus, D. S. et al., 'Red meat-derived heterocyclic amines increase risk of colon cancer: a population-based case-control study', *Nutrition and Cancer*, vol. 65, no. 8, 2013, pp. 1141–50.

53. Alshahrani, S. M. et al., 'Red and processed meat and mortality in a low meat intake population', *Nutrients*, vol. 11, no. 3, 2019.

54. Moss, Michael. *Salt Sugar Fat: How the Food Giants Hooked Us*, New York: Random House, 2013.

55. 'Biology of Food: The Bliss Point', Bloomington: Department of Biology, Indiana University.

56. Achaya, K. T., *Indian Food: A Historical Companion*, New Delhi: Oxford University Press, 1994.

57. Dasgupta, R. et al., 'Sugar, salt, fat, and chronic disease epidemic in India: is there need for policy interventions?', *Indian Journal of Community Medicine*, vol. 40, issue 2, 2015, pp. 71–74.

58. Gulati S. and Misra, 'A: Sugar intake, obesity, and diabetes in India'. Nutrients 6:5955-74, 2014.

59. Dasgupta R. et al., 'Sugar, salt, fat, and chronic disease epidemic in India'.

60. Norat, T. et al., *European Code against Cancer*.

61. Ibid.

62. Mayne, S. T., Playdon, M. C., and Rock, C. L., 'Diet, nutrition, and cancer'.

63. Ibid.

64. Zachariah R: Eating out: Indians cook up $48 billion food business. Mumbai, *The Times of India*, 2013.

65. Ello-Martin JA, Ledikwe JH, Rolls BJ: The influence of food portion size and energy density on energy intake: implications for weight management. Am J Clin Nutr 82:236s-241s, 2005
Paeratakul S, Ferdinand DP, Champagne CM, et al: Fast-food consumption among US adults and children: dietary and nutrient intake profile. J Am Diet Assoc 103:1332-8, 2003
Kushi LH, Doyle C, McCullough M, et al: American Cancer Society Guidelines on nutrition and physical activity for cancer prevention: reducing the risk of cancer with healthy

food choices and physical activity. CA Cancer J Clin 62:30-67, 2012

66. Gulati S, et al., 'Dietary intakes and familial correlates of overweight/obesity: a four-cities study in India', *Annals of Nutrition and Metabolism*, vol. 62, no. 4, 2013, pp. 279–90.

67. O'Keefe, S. J. et al., 'Fat, fibre and cancer risk in African Americans and rural Africans', *Nature Communications*, vol. 6, no. 6342, 2015.

68. Ibid.

69. Crowe, Portia, 'Indians drink way, way more whiskey than Americans', *Business Insider*, 24 June 2015, https://www.businessinsider.com/the-biggest-whiskey-market-in-the-world-2015-6 [accessed: 29 July 2020].

70. Debroyl, S., 'Indians drinking alcohol up 55% in 20 years', *Times of India*, 17 May 2015.

71. Scoccianti, C. et al, 'European Code against Cancer 4th Edition: Alcohol drinking and cancer', *Cancer Epidemioliogy*, vol. 45, 2016, pp. 181–88.

72. GBD 2016 Alcohol Collaborators, 'Alcohol use and burden for 195 countries and territories, 1990-2016: a systematic analysis for the Global Burden of Disease Study 2016', *The Lancet*, vol. 392, pp. 1015–35, 2018.

73. Olds, J. and Milner, P., 'Positive reinforcement produced by electrical stimulation of septal area and other regions of rat brain', *Journal of Comparative and Physiological Psychology*, vol. 47, no. 6, 1954, pp. 419–27.

74. Doyon, W. M. et al., 'Nicotine decreases ethanol-induced dopamine signaling and increases self-administration via stress hormones', *Neuron*, vol. 79, 2013, pp. 530–40.

75. Sharma, R. et al., 'Nicotine administration in the wake-promoting basal forebrain attenuates sleep-promoting effects of alcohol', *Journal of Neurochemistry*, vol. 135, 2015, pp. 323–31.

76.   Blot, W. J. et al., 'Smoking and drinking in relation to oral and pharyngeal cancer', *Cancer Research*, vol. 48, no. 11, 1988, pp. 3282–87.

77.   Scoccianti, C. et al, 'European code against cancer'.

78.   Mayne, S. T., Playdon, M. C., and Rock, C. L., 'Diet, nutrition, and cancer'.

79.   Fortmann, S. P. et al., 'Vitamin and mineral supplements in the primary prevention of cardiovascular disease and cancer: An updated systematic evidence review for the U.S. Preventive Services Task Force'. *Annals of Internal Medicine*, vol. 159, no. 12, 2013, pp. 824–34.

80.   Mayne, S. T., Playdon, M. C., and Rock, C. L., 'Diet, nutrition, and cancer'.

81.   Ibid.

82.   Virtamo J. et al., 'Effects of alpha-tocopherol and beta-carotene supplementation on cancer incidence and mortality: 18-year postintervention follow-up of the Alpha-tocopherol, Beta-carotene Cancer Prevention Study', *International Journal of Cancer*, vol. 135, no. 1, 2014, pp. 178–85.

83.   Neuhouser, M. L. et al., 'Dietary supplement use and prostate cancer risk in the Carotene and Retinol Efficacy Trial', *Cancer Epidemiology, Biomarkers and Prevention*, vol. 18, no. 2, 2009, pp. 2202–06.

84.   Klein, E. A. et al., 'Vitamin E and the risk of prostate cancer: the Selenium and Vitamin E Cancer Prevention Trial (SELECT)', *JAMA*, vol. 306, no. 14, 2011, pp. 1549–56.

85.   Moyer, V. A., 'Vitamin, mineral, and multivitamin supplements for the primary prevention of cardiovascular disease and cancer: U.S. Preventive services Task Force recommendation statement', *Annals of Internl Medicine*, vol. 160, no. 8, 2014, pp. 558–64.

86.   Ibid.

87. Singh et al., 'Global epistemology of obesity, vegetarian dietary patterns, and noncommunicable disease in Asian Indians'.

88. Ibid.

89. Ibid.

90. Ibid.

91. Mehrotra, R. and Singh, K. S., 'Obesity and breast cancer: A wakeup call', *Down to Earth*, 9 May 2019, https://www.downtoearth.org.in/blog/health/obesity-and-breast-cancer-a-wakeup-call-64455 [accessed: 29 July 2020].

92. Singh et al., 'Global epistemology of obesity, vegetarian dietary patterns, and noncommunicable disease in Asian Indians'.

93. Ibid.

94. Ibid.

95. Ibid.

96. Hopkins, B. D., Goncalves, M. D., and Cantley, L. C., 'Obesity and cancer mechanisms: Cancer metabolism', *Journal of Clinical Oncology*, vol. 34, no. 35, 2016, pp. 4277–83.

97. Nagrani, R., et al., 'Central obesity increases risk of breast cancer irrespective of menopausal and hormonal receptor status in women of South Asian Ethnicity', *European Journal of Cancer*, vol. 66, 2016, pp. 153–61.

98. Mayne, S. T., Playdon, M. C., and Rock, C. L., 'Diet, nutrition, and cancer'.

99. Wolin, K.Y. et al., 'Physical activity and colon cancer prevention: a meta-analysis', *British Journal pf Cancer*, vol. 100, no. 4, 2009, pp. 611–16.

100. Eliassen, A. H. et al., 'Physical activity and risk of breast cancer among postmenopausal women', *Archives of Internal Medicine*, vol. 170, no. 19, 2010, pp. 1758–64 and Fournier, A. et al., 'Recent recreational physical activity and breast cancer risk in postmenopausal women in the E3N cohort', *Cancer Epidemiology, Biomarkers and Prevention*, vol. 23, no. 9, 2014, pp. 1893–902.

101. Cheung, L. and Hu, F., 'Examples of moderate and vigorous physical activity', *Obesity Prevention Resource*, Department of Nutrition at Harvard School of Public Health, 2018, https://www.hsph.harvard.edu/obesity-prevention-source/moderate-and-vigorous-physical-activity/ [accessed: 29 July 2020].

102. Bouchard, C., Blair, S. N. and Katzmarzyk, P. T., 'Less sitting, more physical activity, or higher fitness?', *Mayo Clinic Proceedings*, vol. 90, no. 11, 2015, pp. 1533–40.

103. Cuzick, J. et al, 'Prevention and early detection of prostate cancer', *The Lancet: Oncology*, vol. 15, 2014, pp. e484–92.

104. Mayne, S. T., Playdon, M. C., and Rock, C. L., 'Diet, nutrition, and cancer'.

105. Ibid.

106. Anjana, R. M. et al., 'Physical activity and inactivity patterns in India - results from the ICMR-INDIAB study (Phase-1) [ICMR-INDIAB-5]', *International Journal of Behavioral Nutrution and Physical Activity*, vol. 11, no. 1, 2014, p. 26.

107. Schuz, J. et al. 'European Code against Cancer 4th Edition: 12 ways to reduce your cancer risk, *Cancer Epidemioliogy*, vol. 39, suppl. 1, 2015, pp. S1–10.

108. Ibid.

109. Menon, P. et al., 'Trends in Nutrition Outcomes, Determinants, and Interventions in India' (2006-2016), POSHAN Report 10, New Delhi: International Food Policy Research Institute, 2017.

110. Mayne, S. T., Playdon, M. C., and Rock, C. L., 'Diet, nutrition, and cancer' and Kushi, L. H. et al., 'American Cancer Society Guidelines on nutrition and physical activity'.

111. Mayne, S. T., Playdon, M. C., and Rock, C. L., 'Diet, nutrition, and cancer'.

112. American Cancer Society Guideline for Diet and Physical Activity, https://www.cancer.org/healthy/eat-healthy-get-

active/acs-guidelines-nutrition-physical-activity-cancer-prevention/summary.html [accessed: 29 July 2020].

113. Wolfson, J. A. and Bleich, S. N., 'Is cooking at home associated with better diet quality or weight-loss intention?', *Public Health Nutrition*, vol. 18, no. 8, pp. 1397–406, 2015.

114. Panda, A. K. et al., 'New insights into therapeutic activity and anticancer properties of curcumin', *Journal of Exprimental Pharmacology*, vol. 9, 2017, pp. 31–45.

115. Devassy, J. G., Nwachukwu, I. D. & Jones, P. J., 'Curcumin and cancer: barriers to obtaining a health claim', *Nutrition Reviews*, vol. 73, no. 3, 2015, pp. 155–65.

116. Panda, A. K. et al., 'New insights into therapeutic activity and anticancer properties of curcumin'.

117. Ibid.

118. Ibid.

119. See Dhillon, N. et al., 'Phase II trial of curcumin in patients with advanced pancreatic cancer', *Clinical Cancer Research*, vol. 14, no. 14, 2008, pp. 4491–99; Bayet-Robert, M. et al., 'Phase I dose escalation trial of docetaxel plus curcumin in patients with advanced and metastatic breast cancer', *Cancer Biology and Therapy*, vol. 9, no. 1, 2010, pp. 8–14; Kanai, M. et al., 'A phase I/II study of gemcitabine-based chemotherapy plus curcumin for patients with gemcitabine-resistant pancreatic cancer', *Cancer Chemotheraoy and Pharmacology*, vol. 68, no. 1, 2011, pp. 157–64; and Epelbaum, R. et al., 'Curcumin and gemcitabine in patients with advanced pancreatic cancer', *Nutrition and Cancer*, vol. 62, no. 8, 2010, pp. 1137–41.

120. Panda, A. K. et al., 'New insights into therapeutic activity and anticancer properties of curcumin'.

121. Arends, J. et al., 'ESPEN guidelines on nutrition in cancer patients', *Clinical Nutrition*, vol. 36, no. 11, 2016, pp. 11–46.

122. Katz, A. M. and Katz, P. B., 'Diseases of the heart in the works of Hippocrates', *British Heart Journal*, vol. 24, no. 3, 1962, pp. 257–64.

123. Fearon, K. et al., 'Definition and classification of cancer cachexia: an international consensus', *The Lancet: Oncology*, vol. 12, no. 5, 2011, pp. 489–95.

124. Arends, J. et al., 'ESPEN guidelines on nutrition in cancer patients'.

125. Mohan, A. et al., 'High prevalence of malnutrition and deranged relationship between energy demands and food intake in advanced non-small cell lung cancer', *European Journal of Cancer Care*, vol. 26, no. 4, 2016.

126. Ibid.

127. Arends, J. et al., 'ESPEN guidelines on nutrition in cancer patients'.

128. Ibid.

129. Ibid., and National Cancer Institute.

130. Dixon, S., 'Chemotherapy and diet', *Eat Right: Academy of Nutrition and Dietics*, 12 October 2018, https://www.eatright.org/health/diseases-and-conditions/cancer/chemotherapy-and-diet [accessed: 29 July 2020].

131. Ibid.

132. Ibid.

133. Ibid.

134. Ibid.

135. Ibid.

136. Ibid.

137. Terranova, C. O. et al., 'Breast cancer survivors' experience of making weight, dietary and physical activity changes during participation in a weight loss intervention', *Support Care Cancer*, vol. 25, no. 5, 2016, pp. 1455–63.

138. National Cancer Institute.

139. Dixon S, 'Chemotherapy and diet'.

140. Ibid.

141. National Cancer Institute.

142. Ibid.

143. Deng, G. et al., 'Functional magnetic resonance imaging (fMRI) changes and saliva production associated with acupuncture at LI-2 acupuncture point: a randomized controlled study', *BMC Complementary and Alternative Medicine*, vol. 8, no. 37, 2008.

144. Simcock, R. et al., 'ARIX: a randomised trial of acupuncture v oral care sessions in patients with chronic xerostomia following treatment of head and neck cancer', *Annals of Oncology*, vol. 24, no. 3, 2013, pp. 776–83.
      Hovan, A. J. et al., 'A systematic review of dysgeusia induced by cancer therapies', *Support Care Cancer*, vol. 18, no. 8, 2010, pp. 1081–87.

145. Hovan, A. J. et al., 'A systematic review of dysgeusia induced by cancer therapies', *Support Care Cancer*, vol. 18, no. 8, 2010, pp. 1081–87.

146. National Cancer Institute and 'Appetite changes', M. D. Anderson Cancer Center, https://www.mdanderson.org/patients-family/diagnosis-treatment/emotional-physical-effects/appetite-changes.html [accessed: 29 July 2020].

147. Marx, W. et al., 'Chemotherapy-induced nausea and vomiting: A narrative review to inform dietetics practice', *Journal of the Academy of Nutrition and Dietics*, vol. 116, no. 5, 2016, pp. 819–27; Dixon, S., 'Chemotherapy and diet'; and National Cancer Institute.

148. Dixon S., 'Chemotherapy and diet'.

149. Ibid.

150. Ibid.

151. de Cabo, R. and M.P. Mattson, 'Effects of Intermittent Fasting on Health, Aging, and Disease'. *The New England Journal of Medicine*, 2019. 381(26): p. 2541-2551.

152. Demark-Wahnefried, W., et al., 'Feasibility outcomes of a presurgical randomized controlled trial exploring the impact of caloric restriction and increased physical activity versus a wait-list control on tumor characteristics and circulating biomarkers in men electing prostatectomy for prostate cancer'. *BMC Cancer*, 2016, vol. 16, p. 61.

153. de Groot, S., et al., 'Fasting mimicking diet as an adjunct to neoadjuvant chemotherapy for breast cancer in the multicentre randomized phase 2 DIRECT trial'. *Nat Commun.* 2020 Jun 23; 11(1):3083. doi: 10.1038/s41467-020-16138-3. PMID: 32576828; PMCID: PMC7311547.

154. Nencioni, A., et al., 'Fasting and cancer: molecular mechanisms and clinical application'. *Nat Rev Cancer*, 2018. **18**(11): p. 707-719.

155. Ng, A. K. and Travis, L. B., 'Second primary cancers: an overview', *Hematology/Oncology Clinics of North America*, vol. 22, no. 2, 2008, pp. 271–89.

156. Ibrahim, E. M. and Al-Homaidh, A., 'Physical activity and survival after breast cancer diagnosis: meta-analysis of published studies', *Medical Oncology*, vol. 28, no. 3, 2011, pp. 753–65; and Meyerhardt, J. A., Ma, J. and Courneya, K. S., 'Energetics in colorectal and prostate cancer', *Journal of Clinical Oncology*, vol. 28, no. 26, 2010, pp. 4066–73.

157. Ibrahim, E. M. and Al-Homaidh, A., 'Physical activity and survival after breast cancer diagnosis'. *Med Oncol.* 2011 Sep;28(3):753-65. doi: 10.1007/s12032-010-9536-x. Epub 2010 Apr 22. PMID: 20411366.

158. Galvao DA, Taaffe DR, Spry N, et al., 'Combined resistance and aerobic exercise program reverses muscle loss in men

undergoing androgen suppression therapy for prostate cancer without bone metastases: a randomized controlled trial'. J Clin Oncol 28:340-7, 2010.

159. Jones, L. W. et al., 'Effects of an oncologist's recommendation to exercise on self-reported exercise behavior in newly diagnosed breast cancer survivors: a single-blind, randomized controlled trial', *Annals of Behavioral Medicine*, vol. 28, no. 2m 2004, pp.105–13.

160. *Physical Activity Guidelines for Americans*, Washington, DC: US Department of Health and Human Services, 2008.

161. Pinto, B.M. and Ciccolo, J. T., 'Physical activity motivation and cancer survivorship', *Recent Results in Cancer Research*, vol. 186, 2011, pp. 367–87.

162. Peppone, L. J. et al., 'The effect of cigarette smoking on cancer treatment-related side effects', *Oncologist*, vol. 16, no. 12, 2011, pp. 1784–92.

163. O'Malley, M. et al., 'Effects of cigarette smoking on metabolism and effectiveness of systemic therapy for lung cancer', *Journal of Thoracic Oncology*, vol. 9, no. 7, 2014, pp. 917–26.

164. Dhillon, S. et al., 'Risk factors predicting cancer recurrence in lung cancer survivors', *American Journal of Respiratory and Critical Care Medicine*, 2015.

165. Parada H, et al., 'Postdiagnosis changes in cigarette smoking and survival following breast cancer', *JNCI Cancer Spectrum*, vol. 1, no. 1, 2017.

166. Dresler, C. M. et al., 'Reversal of risk upon quitting smoking', *The Lancet*, vol. 368, 2006, pp. 348–49.

167. Kroenke, C. H., et al., 'Weight, weight gain, and survival after breast cancer diagnosis', *Journal of Clinical Oncology*, vol. 23, no. 7, 2005, pp. 1370–78.

168. Rock, C. L. et al., 'Results of the exercise and nutrition to enhance recovery and good health for you (energy) trial: a

behavioral weight loss intervention in overweight or obese breast cancer survivors', *Journal of Clinical Oncology*, vol. 33, no. 28, 2015, pp. 3169–76.

169. Chlebowski, R. T. et al., 'Dietary fat reduction and breast cancer outcome: interim efficacy results from the Women's Intervention Nutrition Study', *Journal of the National Cancer Institute*, vol. 98, no. 24, 2006, pp. 1767–76.

170. Rock C. L., et al, 'Nutrition and physical activity guidelines for cancer survivors', *CA*, vol. 62, no. 4, 2012, pp. 243–74.

171. Demark-Wahnefried, W. et al., 'Changes in weight, body composition, and factors influencing energy balance among premenopausal breast cancer patients receiving adjuvant chemotherapy', *Journal of Clinical Oncology*, vol. 19, no. 9, 2001, pp. 2381–89.

172. Kwan, M. et al., 'Dietary patterns and breast cancer recurrence and survival among women with early-stage breast cancer', *Journal of Clinical Oncology*, vol. 27, no. 6, 2006, pp. 919–26.

173. Meyerhardt, J. A. et al., 'Association of dietary patterns with cancer recurrence and survival in patients with stage III colon cancer', *JAMA*, vol. 298, no. 7, 2007, pp. 754–64.

174. Chlebowski, R. T. et al., 'Dietary fat reduction and breast cancer outcome: interim efficacy results from the Women's Intervention Nutrition Study', *Journal of the Natlional Cancer Institute*, vol. 98, no. 24, 2006, pp. 1767–76.

175. Pierce, J. P. et al., 'Influence of a diet very high in vegetables, fruit, and fiber and low in fat on prognosis following treatment for breast cancer: the Women's Healthy Eating and Living (WHEL) randomized trial', *JAMA*, vol. 298, no. 3, 2007, pp. 289–98.

176. American Institute for Cancer Research, www.aicr.org [accessed: 29 July 2020].

Notes on Contributors

Pushpesh Pant

Pushpesh Pant is a regular recipe columnist and author of many cookbooks in India, including Phaidon's *India: The Cookbook*. He has studied and researched Ayurveda independently for over four decades.

Anita Jaisinghania

A James Beard semifinalist three times for Best Chef Southwest (2012, 2017 and 2018), Anita Jaisinghania's restaurant, Pondicheri in Houton, Texas has been recognized nationwide.

Prasanna Menon

Armed with a PhD in chemistry, Mrs Menon has travelled the world with her Indian diplomat husband. She is a breast cancer survivor and enjoys reading, crafts, bridge and fusion cooking.

Swati Pant

An alumnus of St. Stephen's college in New Delhi and S.P. Jain in Mumbai, Swati Pant is an amateur chef and foodie, and has a deep passion for healthy, low-carb cooking.

Index of Recipes

About the Author

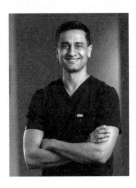

Dr Shubham Pant graduated medical school from Maulana Azad Medical College in New Delhi. He completed his fellowship in Hematology/Oncology from the James Cancer Hospital at The Ohio State University where he was elected Chief Fellow. He served as the Director of Clinical Trials, Section of Hematology/Oncology at the University of Oklahoma.

He is currently an Associate Professor in the Department of Investigational Cancer Therapeutics and the Department of Gastrointestinal Medical Oncology at the University of Texas MD Anderson Cancer Center in Houston, Texas.

Dr Pant is a key opinion leader in the fields of Phase 1 (early drug development) and GI Cancers including pancreatic, biliary, gall bladder and colorectal cancer. He has an expertise in targeted therapy and Immunotherapy and has co-authored numerous peer-review articles. He was recipient of the Mai Eager Anderson Endowed Chair in Cancer Clinical Trials and was featured in '40 under 40' in Oklahoma magazine.

In his free time, Shubham enjoys writing on diet and cancer and is a contributor to Huffington Post and The Quint. He has also anchored health shows on TV including *Living it Up* and *Let's Talk Health*.